Water, Electricity and Health

Protecting ourselves from electromagnetic stress

Alan Hall

HAWTHORN PRESS

Cover design by Ivon Oates
Diagrams by Abigail Large
Typesetting by Hawthorn Press
Printed in the UK by Redwood Books, Wiltshire

British Library Cataloguing in Publication Data applied for

ISBN 1 869 890 94 9

Contents

Contents

Foreword

Christopher Day

Rivetting and informative, this the first book I have seen that brings holistic understanding of how electricity affects life – and what we can do about it.

What do water and electricity have to do with health?

What *are* electricity and water anyway?

Familiar as they are and much as we use them, neither is as simple as it first appears. We know however that electricity is a form of energy and water a receiver and bearer of chemicals, warmth, vibration patterns – and of electricity.

All living things manifest fluidity – in form, growth and substance – and all use, accumulate and release energy. All living things transfer electrical energy within predominantly watery bodies. So fundamental is this that, at a physical level, the harmonious workings of electricity and water are central to health. Health of course is not just an issue of physical substance and simple one-way cause and effect, but nor, as I read from this book, are electricity and water.

We are made of water. About three quarters of our substance, its fluid flow patterns condense to form our organs and shape our bodies. By drinking, eating, breathing and skin exchange, we are constantly exchanging water with our environment – some 15,000 gallons in an average life. No living process can exist without water. No water is without the imprint of micro-structural patterns acquired during its 'biography'. It is these micro-structural patterns, molecular in scale, which can give it life-energising characteristics – and which can be disrupted and distorted by electro-magnetic influences.

The cellular organisation and functioning of the body is regulated by minute electrical signals. At a physical level, living organisms manifest life in electro-chemical terms.

Electricity, magnetism and their electro-magnetic inter-weaving are natural properties of our environment. Birds, insects, even some humans, can navigate in response to magnetic fields 50,000 times weaker than the earth's magnetic field. To put this in context, fields from domestic wiring can be hundreds of thousands of times stronger.

Life on earth has gone on so long we can reasonably assume that electricity and magnetism, as they occur naturally, are, like water, essential to life. But the situation has changed in less than a century, most markedly in barely one generation. The earth's electro-magnetic field, like the human body's, is continually influenced by a host of subtle factors so is ever-varying. Mechanically produced electricity, however, is delivered as alternating current of effectively unvarying wavelength pattern. Whereas living things are in a constant flux of change, lifeless ones endlessly repeat. Unfortunately 'man-made' electro-magnetic fields are thousands of times stronger than natural ones, virtually everywhere – and their oscillations up to several million times more energetic.

Does this have health consequences? This is still a matter of contention – after all there are some *very* financially interested parties. The evidence, however, is increasingly compelling that electro-magnetic fields can be carcinogenic, mutagenic, hormone altering and immunity suppressing.

But this is the world we live in. What can we do about it? Non-ionising electro-magnetic exposure comes from three sources: naturally occurring; wiring and appliances in buildings; power and communications distribution.

Siting buildings near power lines is – or ought to be! – a thing of the past. If they interfere with electronic equipment, think what they do to people! Financial institutions in the US increasingly require electro-magnetic surveys as a condition for mortgages. Some states will not allow new buildings near power lines. In fact, most electro-magnetic exposure originates within buildings – from wiring and appliances.

Man-made electrical and magnetic fields are a recent invention, but electro-magnetic resonances from the earth have been with us from the beginning of time. In the past there was greater sensitivity to such things and building siting often – but not always – intuitively avoided geopathic locations. A study of medieval streets in Regensburg, for instance, showed they followed underground water-courses which intensify and disrupt terrestrial 'radiations' – so preventing houses being built over them.

Grids of electro-magnetic resonance cover the surface of our planet. There are also patterns of intensified energy above geological faults and underground water, both natural and man-made. Where patterns coincide, the energy concentrations can, in the short-term, disrupt sleep and behaviour; in the long-term, lead to serious illness. These patterns can be found by both dowsers and instruments. Ideally buildings should avoid them, but many don't. As with electro-magnetic exposure, the greatest health damage is during sleep. We are in the same position for eight hours and furthermore the body is in cell-repair mode, so particularly vulnerable to disruptive electrical 'signals'. As an architect, I try therefore to ensure beds can never be put in risk locations. Because already built houses are not easy to move, I obstruct bed positions with built-in furniture, doorways and suchlike.

But for these abnormally intense and pattern-disrupted locations, cosmic and terrestrial radiation is natural to life. Indeed it is constantly changing in response to the most delicate cosmic influences – just as living things do. There is every reason to suppose that such radiation – cosmic in origin – is necessary for life. After all, while matter cycles through nature, it is cosmic energy – especially, but not only, that from the sun – that gives it life.

Different building materials obstruct or are permeable by these natural radiations to varying extents. Some plastics are several hundred time more obstructive than natural material alternatives. Extended polystyrene and cork for instance are at opposite ends of the scale of permeability.

Electric fields are relatively easily screened – an advantage with regard to mechanically oscillating ones. The vibrating rhythms of natural electric fields however are 'natural', necessary for healthy life, so much so that NASA found it necessary to artificially generate schumann waves for the health of astronauts. Cages of conductors, such as steel reinforcing rods, electric cable and water pipes can make a sort of 'Faraday cage'. As research on rats has found that living in a Faraday cage leads to sterility in three generations, this is of no small concern. Fortunately, tall apartment blocks have only been common for one human generation and their social consequences (not necessarily unrelated) have already led them into disfavour.

These 'cages' can also carry induced currents, so transporting electro-magnetic fields some distance from their source. In this way different wavelength patterns can interact, intensifying their life-energy disruptive effect.

An electro-magnetic field, like terrestrial radiation, is invisible, but its source is easy to identify. It is a product of electrical *current*, which incidentally, runs in connected cabling even when no appliance is on. Magnetic fields from 2-core cable rotate in opposite directions, so to some extent, cancel each other out. Seperated conductors don't enjoy this benefit, so it is important that conductors for, say, two-way switching, run side by side, best in the same cable. Magnetic fields can be approximately halved by using spiral external-earth cable, earthed metal conduits, or twisted cable (about one twist per foot [30 cm]). Electrical regulations require water-piping to be earthed, but this as connection can transmit induced current, the closer it is to the point the water pipe enters the building, the better.

Most cabling is built in, whereas appliances and furniture get placed at will. Again it is bed positions that are the most critical. Magnetic fields decline with the square of the distance from source, so for most domestic-origin electro-magnetic fields 1.2 metres [4 feet] is usually adequate for safety. Such a distance is relatively easy to plan for if bedside lights are pull-switch controlled. TVs, computers, motors (as in central heating pumps) and transformers (as in fluorescent lights) bring an additional problem. In addition to electro-magnetic fields, these generate vertical columns of disturbance to life-energy. If such a column is crossed by a cable, piping or other conductor, for instance, steel reinforcement, this disharmonic influence can be transmitted long distances. Several sources can interact and intensify this life energy-disrupting effect. No wonder some Building Biologists claim it is unsafe to live above the eighth storey.

It is in fact possible to electrically isolate all cabling when not in use, by using a 'demand switch'. In practice, autonomous appliances like refrigerators, central heating pumps, clocks and the like, should not be included in the rest-of-the-house demand-switched circuit or the whole circuit switches on when they do. Whether they should also be controlled depends on their location and hence the currents and disturbances they induce.

By such means, domestic-origin electro-magnetic field exposure can be minimised and, at health-critical times and locations, effectively eliminated. The problem of non-domestic or non-controllable electro-magnetic fields, however, still remains.

To this, Allan Hall brings another angle of approach. His concern is not electro-magnetic field reduction per se, but to understand and mitigate its effect on life-energy fields – those harmonic resonances emitted by, and nourishing to, all forms of life. Water is the bearer of vibrations, both living and life-less and, at a molecular scale, *all* matter on this earth is coated with a film of water. Vibrational pattern disruptions are in fact much more health-damaging than the electrical and magnetic fields which cause them.

How can life-energy resonance patterns be strengthened and protected from life-less mechanical patterns? This is the subject of this book. It brings the issue of water and its life-supporting characteristics to the fore, and it also leads to a recognition that electricity and magnetism have therapeutic as well as health-damaging potential. This gives a framework of new understanding to electro-biology pioneered some thirty years ago by Robert Becker's work on tissue healing.

Indeed, this approach opens up a whole new way of looking at electricity, water and health.

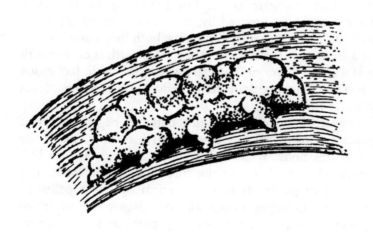

Tardigrada, or Water Bear

Introduction:
A Shifting Balance

Logical thinking cannot yield us any information of the empirical world; all knowledge of reality starts from experience and ends there.

Propositions arrived at by purely logical means are completely empty of reality.

Albert Einstein.

Tardigrada, or the Water Bear, is a very little known but very curious creature. Only a few people have seen one, although they live in large numbers in the sediment in the gutters of your roof, in the damp soil, in ponds and puddles and in many other damp and wet places. The largest is a bit less than one millimeter long, has eight stumpy legs, and spends a lot of its time munching algae. The interesting thing about this creature is what happens to it when algae and water disappear.

When your gutters dry out, the algae die and the water in which the Water Bear thrives evaporates. This would spell disaster for most water creatures, but for the gutter-dwelling Tardigrada this is a common occurrence, for which he has developed a simple survival-strategy. The body of the Water Bear simply dries out to a minute piece of dust, and in this strange sleeping state he does nothing, and just waits for rain. This dehydration can last for a very long time. There is a record of a hundred year-old moss specimen in a museum being placed in water, and a Tardigrada marching out after a century of dehydration. A hundred years is a long time to be without water and yet maintain the vital seed of life.

Water somehow allows life to be expressed.

Familiarity tends to blunt our wonder for this elixir of life. The photographs which were brought back from the first space explorations showed the earth to be incredibly beautiful, as if painted by the hand of a cosmic artist. An ever changing study in blue, white and brown, suspended in an endless ocean of inky black. Alone, fragile, beautiful, delicate. For the first time our whole planet was visible to a human eye from the outside, and this changed people's attitudes to the environment. The blue water of the oceans, the white water of the clouds, both in endless circulation. The earth is a planet on which water is the dominant substance, and in this wonderful womb all life comes to expression.

The earth's wealth of living organisms inhabit only a very thin layer at the surface of the earth, with the majority of species crowding into the soil, the surface of the oceans, and a narrow band of air immediately above them. This spherical shell comprises the Biosphere, or the sphere in which organic life is present. The whole panorama of species in this precious layer, through their absorption and digestion of rocks, each other, sunlight, warmth, air, and so on, act as transformers of the diverse energy systems in, on and above the earth, which are in continual activity and flux. Every clap of thunder, for example, produces nitrogen compounds that are ingested by plants. The sun-drenched tropical ocean generates a current – the Gulf Stream – which flows from the African coast to the Caribbean, then back across the North Atlantic from West to East, to the shores of Northwest Europe. This river of warmth produces an equable but somewhat damp climate, without which this whole region would have very cold winters comparable to those of similar latitude in Labrador in northeast Canada. Or think of a storm-felled tree rotting on the forest floor, providing food for a host of bacteria which transform the wood into new living tissue. Or of the gas reserves trapped in geological strata on the floor of the North Sea since the time when bacteria digested vast tracts of rotting vegetation, which the gas cookers of the UK are now plugged into. Rivers, sunshine, clouds, digestion, heartbeat are all part of the great energy complex of the earth.

To this complex there has now been added a new primary global energy system, that of the electrical power and communications networks.

For long ages, water and life existed in harmonious balance with the natural electrical and magnetic environment of the earth. Now, though, in the twentieth century, exponential growth in the social and industrial use of electricity has occurred almost without question about its environmental impact. There is growing concern amongst individuals, institutions and governments that our new and increasingly indispensable electrical environment is not benign, as has previously been assumed, but is in fact having an effect on life and health. The weight of epidemiological evidence gathered from individual situations increasingly shows that people, animals, plants and ecosystems may all be affected in a variety of ways, some of which may be harmful, and some perhaps beneficial. The situation is, however, extremely complex.

Water is one element in this complex situation which has received comparatively little attention. It forms the major component of all living organisms, and can therefore be singled out as a potentially important part of the puzzle. Indeed, water is the bridge between the silent unseen ocean of electric and magnetic vibrations in which we are now embedded, and the subtle, complex biochemical rhythms that form the foundation of all organic life.

The research work on which the material of this book is based has been carried out at the Live Water Trust in Gloucestershire, UK. This is an independent charity specifically committed to investigating the role of water in the life of the environment under the rapidly changing conditions created by modern society with all its affluence and effluents. This line of investigation has led to a growing concern about the impact that the wide spectrum of twentieth century electromagnetic apparatus is having on the activity of water in large, medium and small ecosystems and organisms.

In order to investigate the interconnections between electromagnetism, water and life in the whole environment, we need to draw on a large number of established scientific disciplines and bodies of knowledge. A study of these complex issues is therefore necessarily interdisciplinary – which in itself poses a challenge to our familiar habits of scientific thought, which always tend to take refuge in narrowly defined fields of research.

Our approach at the Trust has been to identify some of the areas of incompatibility, and to research ways in which these harmful interactions can be transformed. The close co-operation between the nervous system and blood stream in all higher forms of life bears witness to an intimate natural symbiosis between electricity and organic life processes. In principle, therefore, there is no reason why we should not be able to adjust our social use of electricity to be compatible with the general health needs of both the larger and the individual environment. This is the challenge that the emerging problems of the current situation present. Not to reject but to adapt.

Water is a substance that penetrates almost everything – as most seasoned campers have discovered to their cost! As one of the universal media of the organic world, it permeates every organic process in some way, and hence also *integrates* all processes. In this sense, water itself is an interdisciplinary substance. This fact points to the need to study water both in its specific roles in particular situations, and also in its relation to the whole environment. Water has been studied in enormous detail by a veritable army of researchers over the last couple of centuries, and a great deal is known about its properties. Yet despite this enormous volume of work, it still has many enigmatic and poorly understood aspects, particularly its role in the life of organisms.

One of water's properties that we have worked with in some detail, and which is central to the present discussion concerning electricity, is its relation to vibrations. The new ocean of electro-magnetism is an ocean of vibrations, and it is the relation of these to the rhythms of living organisms on which we will concentrate in this book.

To move into the realm of *life* is to move into a region where measurement of quantity has less value than in the exact world of electromagnetism, where so much has been achieved through precise, quantitative measurement. The functioning of the TV is so bewilderingly complex that its technical success could only have been achieved through exact observation and highly disciplined calculation.

Our own health, on the other hand, cannot be quantified in the same way. The fact that we cannot exactly measure our sense of well-being, however, does not in any way deny the reality of our experience. We all experience hope and despair, which are intensely real – yet there is no standard scale to measure them by: we may speak of utter despair or great hope, but not of 85.3 percent despair! The whole medical profession relies on reports of how patients feel, and there are as many diverse patterns of experience as there are individuals. When we consider the imponderable, fluctuating element of our experience of life, we are not entering into someone else's specialist area – it is our own, personally valid domain, which nobody can quantify.

So in trying to find an understanding of the relationship between the two very different worlds of electromagnetism and life, there is at the outset a potential conflict between the *methodology* of investigation into the two realms. One relies heavily on the capacity to measure and quantify, which is inimical to the other. The unique experience of each individual is valid, even if the apparent objectivity of an electrical instrument's digital read-out can find no use for it.

We certainly do not claim to have solved the problems that this dichotomy creates, but we have worked from 'both ends', which has led to quite definite results. One is to identify new aspects of the action of electromagnetism in the environment. The second is to find new practical means to overcome some of the harmful effects of electromagnetism on people and other organisms. Simply *avoiding* exposure to such influences is increasingly difficult and not a real solution.

This work is only at the beginning, and raises many questions which remain unanswered. We will discuss a number of apparently unrelated topics in order to throw some light on the complexities of the relation between electricity and life. Our health is intimate, it is ours and we care about it, yet we know very little about ourselves. Electricity is 'out there', well understood in engineering terms, and yet remains completely enigmatic; we do not know its real nature, and have no sense for it. So it is hardly surprising that opinions are sharply divided on issues concerning the relationship between the two. In such a situation it is wise to consider as much evidence and as many relevant points of view as possible.

This book has not been written for the specialist, but is intended to be accessible to everyone. It gives the results of research from a totally different perspective from that used in most studies and laboratories, drawing on concepts which, if taken seriously, could help shed some light on this difficult but vital subject. There is at present great public concern about the health risks of electricity use, but it is not our aim to fuel this concern, so much as to address the problems and seek solutions.

Electricity, magnetism, water and life are four diverse elements which all form vital ingredients of our natural environment, and have done so for geological ages. Now, in the late twentieth century, the balance between them is very rapidly changing. In the following pages we will look at some of the causes and effects of this shift, and at possible solutions and remedies for what has become a problem of far-reaching dimensions.

Chapter 1:
A Sea of Trouble: The New Electromagnetic Ocean

Even though we now know that things which are invisible and imperceptible to us are not necessarily harmless, (e.g. radioactivity and X-rays), electricity has become such a central part of our lives that it is hard to question its unseen effects. Yet evidence of its potential danger to health is continually accumulating, and can no longer be disregarded.

The Simmonds family moved into a new house in rural Gloucestershire in 1985. They had two sons, Malcolm aged 10, and Peter aged 5. The previous owners had sold following a series of problems including depression. Peter was a sensitive child and had suffered from slight chest problems before moving, but nothing serious. Soon after moving in, both boys became unwell. Peter, particularly, suffered from very severe asthma. He also found it almost impossible to sit in the kitchen at any time. Both Mr. and Mrs. Simmonds, who both spent a good deal of time at home with their work, began to feel permanently tired and exhausted.

Peter's white blood count was very high, but doctors could not identify any specific illness. He often cried, could not stand the water in the bath, and often complained that he couldn't control his thoughts. His words also became muddled and confused. Mr. Simmonds would sometimes black out while working at his desk, even first thing in the morning. The family became desperate, feeling caught in some unidentified downward spiral. After a 7-year saga involving various advisors, treatments and considerable expense, the source of the problem was identified. There was an overhead power cable about 300 yards from the house, and running under both the cable and the house was an underground stream. The kitchen was directly over the waterflow. The family eventually moved, everyone's health improved, and Peter is now a competent student of the sciences.

This by no means unique example shows how the electrical energy system that we all use can indirectly have a powerful effect on our general health. A huge amount of research into the effects of electricity on health has been done over the last fifteen years (see bibliography) and while expert and professional opinion is sharply divided over the findings, many scientists are extremely concerned.

Professor Ross Adey of the Loma Linda University Medical School in California has been researching the effects of electricity on the living world for over 30 years. He was previously Director of the NASA Space Biology Institute, Professor of Anatomy and Physiology UCLA, founder of UCLA Brain Research Institute, and a member of the Academy of Science Committee studying the biological effects of the military Seafarer Extra Low Frequency Communications System. In 1992, in a programme for BBC Radio Scotland, he spoke about the possible adverse health effects of electric fields created typically by electrical power that everyone uses.

As far as the science itself goes, I think that there are four major areas about which there can be little doubt as to the significance of the findings:

1. The effects on the immune system. A reduction in the ability of the circulating white blood cells to kill tumor cells. This has been shown in cell culture work and partially corroborated in animal studies.

2. Effects on foetal development. There is evidence not only from abnormalities but also in psycho-sexual development. Epidemiological work has shown that

miscarriages may be linked to electric blanket use and some electrical home heating.

3. The area of the control and regulation of cell growth, including tumor formation.

4. The effects on the central nervous system and the brain in ways which affect very powerful hormonal mechanisms, which in turn have connections to cancer and cancer-related problems.

[...] I think that the British authorities' reaction is a living dinosaur attitude, that it absolutely avoids confronting the evidence as it now exists. The NRPB, (National Radiological Protection Board), however, is doing work of the highest merit in its scientific content, and it indicates that there is reason for concern. [1]

The National Radiological Protection Board published a report in March 1992, which specifically addressed the issue of cancer risk from electromagnetic fields:

The greatest concern has been caused by the reports of an excess cancer in children who have been exposed to above average levels of electromagnetic fields by virtue of their place of residence. Seven studies have been reported since the appearance of the first in 1979, all of a case control type, in which comparisons have been made between the proximity of various sources of electromagnetic fields to the places of residence of children who had or had not developed cancer. The results have been variable, but taken at face value, they appear to provide some weak evidence of support of the postulated association [...]

The results of some of the whole animal and cellular studies suggest the possibility that electromagnetic fields might act as co-carcinogens or tumor promotors but, taken overall, the data are inconclusive... [2]

It has proved very difficult to establish a clear causal relationship between known electromagnetic environments and specific effects and disorders. Clarity is confounded by the large number of interrelated variable factors that work in any living system. This difficulty in establishing clear cause-effect diagnosis is due mainly to two factors. First, a lack of understanding of long-term effects of the interaction between the apparently disparate entities of electromagnetism and living organisms. Second, our tendency to think in terms of a single cause for a single effect.

Although connections may appear elusive, this does not automatically imply that electromagnetism is not involved as a factor in certain well-known disorders in health. The case history evidence tends to suggest that it is.

Just a few typical examples of the research work, evidence, and individual cases are given below. Most effects are due to three primary sources of disturbance: i) the 50 or 60Hz electrical power system and its apparatus; ii) the broadcast radio frequency transmissions; and iii) individual pieces of equipment, such as computers.

i) Effects on health of 50/60 cycle mains power supplies and apparatus

The number of government agency investigations into this area indicates a growing concern about the interaction of people and electrical systems.

In America the EPA (Environmental Protection Agency), which is roughly equivalent to the UK Ministry of the Environment, produced an internal draft report in 1990, titled *Evaluation of the Potential Carcinogenicity of Electromagnetic fields.*[3] This report was never officially published, even though the investigation found enough evidence of a causal link between electromagnetic fields in domestic situations and the incidence of cancers, particularly in children, to recommend that electromagnetic fields should be included on the list of class B1 carcinogens. This appears to be a clear though unofficial assessment of the possible risks to health involved in the use of electrical systems.

In Sweden in 1982, Dr. Kjell Hanson Mild, working for the National Board of Occupational Safety and Health, published a review of neurophysiological effects of electromagnetic radiation, and quoted no fewer than 3,627 research articles in the world scientific literature at that time which showed a connection between electromagnetic fields and living processes. [4]

In 1994 the Swiss Federal Department of the Environment published a report by a medical commission on the biological effects of extra low frequency (50Hz) electromagnetic fields. They found that 'the causal link between electromagnetic fields and cancer has been convincingly demonstrated' (by current research).[5]

The Fishponds Case

Fishponds is a tiny village in Dorset, UK, over which a new 275kV and 400kV power grid line was erected in 1967 (1Kv=1,000volts). Only after a delay of six years did this group of people living in a very quiet and beautiful valley find that they began to develop a number of new and unusual symptoms. As this is a very well documented and geographically isolated situation, the full details are very instructive. There were 19 houses all within one mile of the cable. The numbers refer to individual houses shown on the map in **diagram 1**.[6]

1. Previous history of hypertension, retired early from merchant navy; very sudden heart-attack death after working all weekend in part of garden of no. 7, directly under cables. Visitors reported sleeplessness and dizziness.

2. Petit-mal epilepsy in adolescent boy, now controlled by medication. Later, severe exhaustion illness in very lively mother.

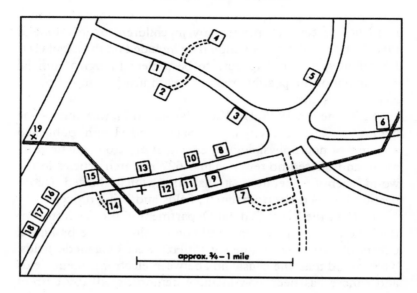

Diagram 1: Map of Fishponds village, in Dorset

3. Rare cancer of eye; eye removed. Bees swarm unusually angrily.

4. Very severe heart condition, considerably relieved on leaving the village.

5. Sleeplessness due to howling and throbbing of the lines.

6. Holiday home, but vet advised owner not to leave donkey in field directly under lines. Night-light continues to burn after being turned off.

7. Two separate cases of black-outs; one grand-mal epilepsy, food allergies, rashes, raised leucocyte (white blood cell) count; sleeplessness, exhaustion, headaches, depression, muscular weakness.

8. Dizziness, some loss of muscle strength when outside.

9. One unexpected heart-attack death, following a history of one-sided headaches and persistent skin rashes; one case of recurrent severe heart palpitations; strong asthmatic reaction in daughter whenever visiting.

10. Severely swollen limbs, with muscular distress and pain in joints; dizziness, sleeplessness.

11. Previous serious heart condition severely aggravated immediately on moving to village, death within a few months.

12. Original family: one cancer, which improved on leaving the village. Nervous tension needing medication, dizziness, severe eye strain and drying up of retinal fluid in one eye. Grandchild who visited frequently developed skin rashes when sleeping in pram under lines, later petit-mal epilepsy. Second family: former electrical engineer with heart trouble died suddenly of heart-attack shortly after returning from two months holiday. Sleeplessness due to throbbing sensation throughout body.

13. One case of black-out, together with frequent dizziness and occasional total loss of muscle power (i.e. collapse), even though inside the house. Severe headaches for all the family. Very unusual and severe rash in small child, which baffled the specialist.

14. Cancer leading to hysterectomy; eye strain, headaches.

15. No symptoms reported, but two new TV sets blew up in succession.

16. Dizziness, heart palpitations, headaches, near-clinical depression. Bees kept near lines became aggressive and stopped making honey until taken 20 miles away, at the advice of the Bee Inspector.

17. Holiday home, little used; but visiting friend fell off moped due to black-out under lines, broke ribs.

18. Two cataracts, removed in middle age.

19. Well known dangerous accident spot (several fatal).

This situation developed into a test case with the distribution authority, who at that time denied any causal link between the various symptoms of illness and the power line, despite the fact that out of a total of 30 permanent residents, 23 reported either non-specific or clinical symptoms of illness. It also shows the effects of chronic exposure and the time delay between exposure and the onset of an illness. The line was installed in 1967, and the data above dated from 1987. The problem remains unresolved. This chronic and cumulative effect is a common feature of all health problems related to low level, chronic electromagnetic field exposure, well known in the band of ionising radiations, such as the far-ultra violet (UV band C), and X-rays.

Damages claims on personal health and property devaluation grounds are being pursued in several countries (including the UK), between individuals and various agencies who handle electrical supply and distribution. In America in 1985 a private school group sued the Houston Lighting and Power company for increasing the risk of cancer to school children due to the installation of high voltage power lines across the school area. They won the case, and damages of $25.1 million were awarded against the power company, even though no one had fallen ill. The award was made on the grounds of **potential health risk.**

Nancy Wertheimer, an epidemiologist in America who made one of the early studies of childhood and adult cancer, found correlations with the layout of electrical power distribution cables. In 1979 she published a report [7] on a study of a total of 494 cases of death from childhood leukaemia in the Denver area. Later she worked on a further case control study of 1,179 cases of adult mortality from cancer. These studies showed a higher incidence of cancer amongst adults and children living in houses close to high-current distribution cables. Her work was initially more or less ignored, despite being published in the highly respected American Journal of Epidemiology which is published by the John Hopkins University School of Hygiene and Public Health. As more evidence began to accumulate in the 1980s, her research began to be viewed in a new light. She wrote in the opening paragraph of her original report:

> Electrical power came into use many years before environmental impact studies were common, and today our domestic power lines are taken for granted and generally assumed to be harmless. However, this assumption has never been adequately tested. Low-level harmful effects could be missed, yet they might be important for the population as a whole, since electric wires are so ubiquitous. In 1976-1977, we did a field study in the greater Denver area which suggested that, in fact, the homes where children developed cancer were found unduly often near electric lines carrying high currents.

ii) Effects to health of radio, TV, and radar transmissions

During the Cold War period, the American government maintained an embassy in Moscow. In 1976 the United States accused the Soviet authorities of directing very high-frequency microwave radio waves (2.5-4.0 GHz, one GHz being one thousand million cycles per second) at the embassy. The Soviets denied it, but measurements proved it to be a fact. Much later it was found that the US State Department knew all about the radiation back in 1953, but chose not to disclose it. The effects of this radiation on the embassy staff have only emerged slowly through a fog of confusion, and on the basis of around 2,500 documents released under the Freedom of Information Act. There were a variety of disorders which show a high incidence in the embassy staff, such as eye problems, psoriasis, skin disorders, depression, irritability, loss of appetite, and difficulty in concentrating. Children living in the building showed abnormal levels of anaemic blood diseases, mumps, heart disease and respiratory infections. Several diplomats developed leukaemia, and two of the three US ambassadors in the peak period of 1953-77 died of cancer; the third died of leukaemia, which was first discovered in 1975 when he was taken ill with nausea and bleeding. This is a classic and rather dramatic example, and it should be noted that the power level of this radiation was around $5\mu W/cm^2$. The official American safety standard for microwave radiation is $50mW/cm^2$, but the Russian standard is $10\mu W/cm^2$, which is *a 1000 times lower;* and the embassy radiation was *half* of this lower safe limit (One mW = $1,000\mu W$). This posed a dilemma for the US Government, and, as a consequence, there have been several out-of-court settlements to embassy personnel who sued for damages on health grounds.

There are many research papers about the interaction of radio frequency and microwave frequency radiations. For example, Bob Lidburdy, researching into bioelectromagnetics at Lawrence Berkley in America, found as long ago as 1979 that such radiation affected the blood T- and B-cell levels, as well as causing a reduction in the immune system function.[8] Other researchers have confirmed connections between low-level radio frequency fields and immune system disorders.

A Polish scientist, Dr. Stanislaw Szmigielski, is known internationally, and respected for his work on the effects of radio and microwave radiation on the immune system. He has produced preliminary results from studying military personnel which show a correlation between microwave radiations and certain forms of cancer. Military personnel exposed to radio and micro-wave radiation were seven times more likely to develop cancers in organs involving blood formation and lymphatic tissue.[9] Exposure times of those investigated varied from 5 to 15 years.

Portable telephone systems

The past few years have seen an explosion in the use of mobile phones. These work at high radio frequencies and require for their operation a country-wide network of aerials and radio transmitter-receivers. In the UK the planning law has been flouted in order to make way for this.

The latest development in America is 'Personal Communications Systems' or PCS, which are designed to work at higher frequencies with more advanced technology, to allow the network to handle data and information transfer. These work at 1.9GHz, which is close to that of microwave ovens at 2.4GHz. This means that this frequency is transmitted over the whole area of cover 24 hours a day – whether you are using a phone or not. Some 100,000 aerials are planned in America in order to achieve complete coverage, and this will create a permanent electromagnetic ocean of this 1.9GHz frequency. The industry plans to make this a global system within the next few years.

There are serious concerns about the health effects of very low-level radiation of this sort of frequency. Following the inauguration of this new system in New York, quite a large number of electrically sensitive people suddenly began to suffer from serious stress-symptoms. These included eye problems, dry lips, pains in the chest, insomnia, dizziness and nausea. Moving away from the area seemed to be the only solution for these people.

The power levels of the new electromagnetic fields are very low unless you are using a phone – but low-level does *not* necessarily mean safe. The key principle applied in the regulation of any chemical toxin, such as nitrates in drinking water, is that there is a concentration level below which it is considered safe to ingest it. This approach has led to the assumption that the 'low is safe' principle can be applied equally to any and all environmental pollution, including radio frequency radiation. Yet, as electrically sensitive people demonstrate, research points towards the cumulative effects of long-term, low-level exposure, and even suggests that we may be *more* sensitive to low levels than to higher ones. Such findings seriously challenge the wisdom of plunging everyone into this new ocean, without even allowing them any choice in the matter.

iii) Individual equipment

Computer screens and TVs emit a range of radiations. The effect of computer terminals on health is well documented in the book *Terminal Shock*.[10] Problems are reported from many countries, particularly amongst pregnant women who spend time in front of a screen. In Japan, for example, a survey of 13,000 computer operators, of whom 4,500 were women, showed that a total of 250 of them had become pregnant or given birth during the survey. 36 per cent (91) had abnormal pregnancies which included 8 miscarriages, 8 premature births, and 5 stillbirths, with a high correlation between abnormal pregnancy and high exposure times. Other commonly reported problems are deformities and low birth-weight. Similarly, a study in California of some 1500 pregnant women working on computer terminals, showed a roughly 100 per cent increase in miscarriages.[11]

The above examples are only a small sample chosen to give some idea of just how much is known about this complex issue, for those readers who are not at all familiar with the subject. The effects of electromagnetic stress on people are so complex because there are five key interacting elements.

1. The presence of vibrating electric, electromagnetic and magnetic fields.

2. Field vibrations over a wide frequency range.

3.   The individual's medical biography.

4.   Exposure times and intensities.

5.   Interaction with other factors such as physical pollutants.

These five interrelated elements in any one individual's situation make it difficult to be clear about what set of conditions precipitate which symptoms and eventual illnesses. This is compounded by an individual moving about in the normal course of daily life between different places where stress levels vary.

One thing is clear. Exposure to quite low levels of any or all of the three fields over long periods of time, can cause serious debilitating decline in a range of body functions.

Stress of any sort such as worry, uncertainty, overwork or poor diet, makes us vulnerable to opportunistic infections and illnesses connected with inherent weaknesses. We are not normally aware of the three fields which cause electromagnetic stress, and when chronic symptoms of unease or minor illness occur, the cause often remains unidentified. Such conditions may continue for years, as in the case of the Simmonds family quoted above, causing much unnecessary suffering and expense.

The main functional areas that appear to be affected are the immune response system, concentration, formation of thoughts, memory, digestion, breathing and heart rhythms. There are, of course, many disorders that signal symptoms in any of these areas, and such disorders can have a multitude of causes. The effect of the electromagnetic environment is only *one* possible cause of disorder, which may act alone, or together with other stresses, infections and weaknesses.

The medical aspects of these stress-related illnesses is an area for the medical profession. Our concern at The Live Water Trust is not to encroach upon this medical field, but to help raise awareness of two issues:

- Electromagnetic stress is often an unrecognised and undiagnosed factor in many minor and serious illnesses, including slow recovery from illness.

- There are ways in which electromagnetic stress can be reduced or eliminated.

Experiences from a range of specific situations show the following early warning symptoms which may indicate that individuals are suffering from the effects of electromagnetic stress:

Low energy levels
Lowering of concentration
Reduced memory function
Difficulty in thinking
Persistent headaches
Depression
Dizziness
Allergic reactions
Breathing difficulty
Frequent minor illnesses such as colds and flu
Slow recovery from minor illnesses
Hyperactivity in children
Disturbed or shallow sleep
General exhaustion
Loss of appetite
Muscular weakness
Irritability

There is very strong evidence that specific illnesses and serious disorders are caused or exacerbated by long term exposure to electromagnetic stress. Such conditions include:

Eye cataracts
Soft tissue cancers
Birth deformities

Skin rashes
Black-outs
Leukaemia
Miscarriages
Heart strain
Immune deficiencies

The evidence to support the view that the electromagnetic ocean is having a harmful effect on our health is becoming ever stronger. We now need to examine its relationship to the ecosystems of the earth, and to water in particular.

---

[1] Professor Ross Adey, on Speaking out, BBC Radio Scotland, 10 January 1992

[2] NRPB 'Doll' Report, March 1992

[3] EPA/600/6-90/0058

[4] Kjell Hansson Mild and P.A. Oberg, 1982: Neurophysiological Effects of Electromagnetic Fields; a Critical Review, Kyoto Symposia (EEG suppl. no. 36).

[5] Swiss Federal Department of the Environment, 1994

[6] Cyril Smith and Simon Best, 1989: Electromagnetic Man, Health and Hazard in the Electrical Environment, J.M. Dent and Sons, London.

[7] Wertheimer N., Leeper E., 1979: 'Electrical wiring configurations and childhood cancer' in the *American Journal of Epidemiology* 109-273-284. Also, Wertheimer N., Leeper E., 1982: 'Adult cancer related to electrical wires near the home' in *Bioelectromagnetics* 9:195-205.

[8] R. Lidburdy, 1979: 'RF radiation alters the immune system; modulation of T and B lymphocyte levels and cell-mediated immunocompetence by hyperthermic radiation' in *Radiation Research 77*.

[9] Stanislaw Szmigielski et al: *Immunologic and Cancer-related Aspects of Exposure to Low-level Microwave and Radio Frequency Fields*, Swiss Federal Department of the Environment 1994.

[10] Bob de Matteo, 1986: *Terminal Shock: The Health Hazard of VDUs*, N.C. Press, Toronto.

[11] Goldhaber G., Polen M., Hiatt R.: 'Risk of miscarriage and birth defects among women who use video display terminals during pregnancy' in the *American Journal of Independent Medicine 13*, 695-706.

Chapter 2:
Vibration and Rhythm

We live in an ocean of air. The oxygen from this ocean penetrates every cell of our body when we breathe – a most sophisticated process that regulates the flow of oxygen into, and the flow of carbon dioxide out of our lungs. For most of our life we are not conscious of this natural regulation, unless we focus our attention on it or are afflicted by some form of temporary or chronic crisis. An imbalance in this vital breathing process immediately affects us, warning that something is wrong.

The ocean of air from which we draw our breath covers the entire planet to a height of some twelve miles or so, becoming rarer the higher we go. It is self-evident that both we and the whole biosphere are dependent upon this ocean. Although all organisms depend on the air, the process varies from one type of organism to another. All the higher life-forms take oxygen from the air as they breathe in, and add carbon dioxide as they breathe out. The plants do the same at night, but during the day, under the influence of sunlight, the reverse is the case. Through photosynthesis, water is broken down, hydrogen used to build sugars, and the surplus oxygen transpired to the air. If this did not happen, the oxygen in the air would soon be used up; and so a delicate balance is achieved in the atmosphere between supply and demand, both of oxygen and carbon dioxide. The whole biosphere is extremely delicately adjusted to the chemical energy system of the air. Our current concern about global warming is in part due to the vulnerability of this delicate balance, for very small changes in the carbon dioxide levels can become amplified and start to have a major effect on the atmosphere, the biosphere, the sea-currents and so on.

We are surrounded and filled with vibrations and rhythms. Some of these affect us consciously, but the majority flow below the threshold of our waking life. Some, like sound, give us joy; others, such as the heaving deck of a boat, can generate deep disturbance; some, like radioactivity, are so far removed from our awareness that we cannot sense them at all.

Bird song, human speech, and music all generate vibrations in the air and in everything that the air touches. We do not usually have a direct experience of the air moving, except when the bass section of an orchestra or band really gets going. Yet, when the chaffinch sings its dawn song, it sets the air into delicate vibration for hundreds of yards around, like a large, very mobile jelly being carefully shaken. The pattern of shaking is so finely sculpted that it is possible to recognise the call of the chaffinch amidst all the other birds competing for our attention. A very well-tuned ornithologist's ear can even detect a difference between birds of differing localities. The chaffinch has a two-part call; the first phrase is universal to the species wherever it lives. The second is a local 'dialect' belonging only to chaffinches of a particular district. On tape recordings this can be analysed quite exactly, just as surely as we can recognise a local accent in a friend's voice. Sound, then, affects us at a conscious level, through the organ in us which is tuned to the reception of such vibrations – the ear.

The air carries towards us a vast range of different vibrations, all with their own nuances and subtle variations. It is quite rare to find a place where the air is quite still, and to experience complete silence. If the air vibrates at a frequency anywhere between about 20 and 20,000 times a second, then we experience sound of a particular pitch.

There is a limit to the pitch of sound that we can hear, which varies from person to person depending on age, amount of damage incurred through exposure to loud noise, and congenital factors. The typical upper limit of a healthy young adult is around the 20,000 cycles per second mentioned above. Above this frequency we are not likely to hear anything. However, the Hi-Fi recording industry has discovered that if frequencies above 20,000 are left out of music-recordings, a critical ear can still detect a difference. Including these frequencies improves the quality of the sound. This is a very interesting fact which points to the importance of the whole fabric of the frequencies. We apparently have a sense for the whole, even though we do not, in this case, have a specific sense for all the vibrations which compose it.

The oceans are not silent either. The longest coherent animal call in nature comes from the whales. One single series of expressions can last for half an hour without any repeating phrases. These very evocative sounds set the water vibrating rather than the air, and by using layers of water that are at a constant temperature, the whale can transmit these vibrations for hundreds of miles across the ocean, which preserves the integrity of the vibrating pattern so that the sound can be heard by a fellow whale or a submerged microphone. In this way a huge body or 'tube' of water is set vibrating in a highly structured but very transient form.

Trains, aircraft and cars never give us a smooth journey, whatever the advertisers say: everything vibrates. Leave the window open a couple of inches or so in some types of car, and a very low-frequency throbbing vibration can be set up which can lead to serious discomfort or even vomiting. Our abdomen can be stimulated by frequencies around 6-7Hz, well below our threshold of sound-perception, so travel sickness can be triggered by vibrations.

Our brain functions in an atmosphere of vibrations, ranging from around 1/4Hz for the breathing mediated through the cerebro-spinal fluid, to 1.2Hz for the blood pulse, to 8-30Hz in the nervous tissues. Our muscles carry a background vibration, or muscle 'tone' during waking hours. Some species of moth vibrate their wings at particular frequencies, modulating their radiating infra-red body heat in order to attract a mate of the same species. Over a mile away, a male moth can detect the mechanical frequency of the female's wings, transferred to the infra-red radiation which it can sense through its antennae. This is a common mode of communication among insects which are highly tuned to particular frequencies in individual organs, such as antennae.[1] Bees have evolved a very sophisticated language of communication: through vibrations of their abdomens they communicate the direction, distance and quality of a particular source of nectar to other bees in the colony.[2]

Seismographic records show a constant stream of vibrations coming from the earth, bearing witness to the titanic forces driving the tectonic plates against each other under the continents and oceans. Only when these reach dramatic proportions during earthquakes do we become aware of their existence. The earth is quaking all the time, but we fail to notice its subtler energy changes. Lorries, cars, trains, waterfalls and the ocean's waves on the shore all add local components to these natural background disturbances. These are just a few examples of vibrations of physical substances, both mineral and organic. Such patterns of movement, being physical, are usually accessible either directly, or through fairly simple instruments, and form one class of vibrations in which we are embedded, and through which we participate in the world of tangible things.

We also inhabit an ocean of electricity, and another of magnetism. Like the air, these form a vital part of our natural environment and have done so since the dim and distant past. We and other organisms have evolved in harmony with these other two invisible oceans, just as surely as we have evolved with the ocean of air. They penetrate us day and night, but we normally have no direct sense of their presence, their benefits or the harm that they may cause. Unlike our breathing, of which we are at least unconsciously aware, we do not appear to have any immediate capacity for regulating our exposure to the forces of magnetism and electricity. These forces are quite different from mechanical vibrations, for no physical substance needs to move when they vibrate. Yet they still affect many physical substances – water being one – and need physical substance for their genesis.

Until recent time, these oceans of electricity and magnetism were either unknown or largely ignored, except perhaps for an interest in the violence of thunderstorms, and in compass-guided global navigation. 150 years ago in 1844, this situation began to change when Samuel Morse, of code fame, installed the first pair of wires to carry electricity between Baltimore and Washington in America, creating the first practical electrical communication system on the earth. The first commercial step in creating a global electrical power distribution system was the opening of the Holborn Viaduct power station, London, which sold its first unit of electricity to a consumer on 12 January 1882.

Since these first modest beginnings, *billions* of miles of wire have been spun around the globe in the most mind-bendingly complex and precise patterns, to create our modern communications and electrical power systems.

This electrical web now forms a major *new* energy system on the earth. Such an energy system, though, is not isolated but forms a part of all the other interacting global energy systems, large and small. Some effects of introducing this new system are obvious, such as electricity pylons striding across the country-side and the enormous social changes that electricity has brought about, while others are less so – like the effects on health.

So man has, in various ways, harnessed these non-physical vibrations. One example of the creation of such 'non-physical movement' very relevant to the present discussion, is the use, and the reason for using, three-phase electrical power – both nationally in the UK and world-wide. This system of power generation and distribution is the brain-child of one man, the Croatian Nikola Tesla, who emigrated to America in his twenties. After finishing his university studies and before leaving Europe, he was in Budapest, and had become obsessed with solving the problem of the inherent deficiencies of the early electric motors of the middle to late nineteenth century. He had drastically overworked himself, and fell ill to the point of near-death. He recovered slowly, and while convalescing was one day walking with a friend, Szigety, in a park in Budapest at sunset, reciting Goethe's Faust – which, having a photographic memory, he knew by heart:

> *The glow retreats, done is the day of toil:*
> *It yonder hastes, new fields of life exploring:*
> *Ah, that no wings can lift me from the soil,*
> *Upon its track to follow, follow soaring.*
>
> *A glorious dream, though now the glories fade.*
> *Alas, the wings that lift the mind no aid*
> *Of wings to lift the body can bequeath me.*[3]

At this point he stopped in his tracks, and exclaimed, 'I can see it'. The gestation period had been long and very painful; the inspiration came in a flash. Szigety thought his friend had lapsed into his previous delirium, but Tesla, endowed with an incredibly vivid and accurate imagination, could quite literally see the solution to the problem he had struggled with – how to improve the efficiency of the electric motor. In one moment of inspiration he created the three-phase electrical system.

As with most brilliant ideas, his was absurdly simple. He saw three coils of wire, arranged as in **diagram 2**, and three separate electrical supplies which all vibrated – an entirely new idea at this time (around 1882). The germinal electrical industry was using supplies that were steady, like any battery. Tesla imagined three vibrating supplies, all with the same frequency, but not all synchronised, rather like a twelve-bar round in music in which three groups sing the identical notes and melody, but each starts four bars behind the other. If the timing of each group is accurate, then harmony is achieved. Three phase power supplies all vibrate at 50Hz, but each supply is out of time with the other two by an exact amount. This is what Tesla saw. The result is very remarkable. The three coils of wire in the diagram are fixed in space; they do not move. In the interior space they create a magnetic field which rotates 3000 times a minute. Nothing physical moves, but a magnetic field is generated with perpetual rotation.

If a bar of iron is put into this field it will spin round, drawn by the magnetism. This is the basis of the majority of industrial electric motors to this day. They are very efficient, and require very little maintenance. This is the basic reason for electric pylons carrying cables in sets of three.

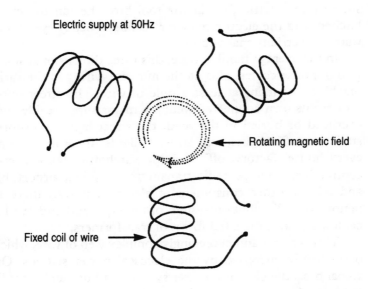

Diagram 2: Creating a rotating magnetic field
with stationary coils of wire

But to return to our domestic use of electricity, just imagine, for a moment, your home without the walls, floors, ceilings, furniture, and any of the physical aspects of the house *except* the electrical wires, and the pieces of iron round which some of them are closely wrapped in tight coils, in the washing-machine motor for example. Just begin to tot it all up. First there is the mains house-wiring in every room, to the lights and the power sockets – about half a mile of wire. Then there are all the various pieces of electrical equipment, such as the vacuum cleaner, fridge, freezer, washing machine, stove, central heating pump and controls, food mixer, microwave cooker, fluorescent lights, TV, radio, CD player, video recorder, and the electric fire. Then there are the communications devices, such as telephone, fax, burglar alarm and security systems. You probably also have a doorbell system, and various machines such as an electric drill in the tool box, the fan to vent the kitchen, and the electricity meter keeping a beady eye on every watt of electricity that you use.

In the average family house, this three dimensional spider's web of house cables, plus all the intricate wiring in the various machines, contains at least a mile of wire. The street outside also has its own connected web; the mains supply cable, either overhead or buried in the road, the street lights, transformer stations, traffic lights, and street bollards. In order to supply every house, factory, office, shop, warehouse, school, leisure centre, farm, college, radio transmitter, hospital, airport, bank and all the other consumers of electrical power, there is a nation-wide distribution system of underground and overhead cables, and an associated forest of transformers.

This is a vast and exceedingly complex web of wire, which is permanently energised by the electrical power stations. On a global basis the electrical power system is a huge and incredibly engineered energy system, with a highly sophisticated infrastructure. It is a credit to human ingenuity and industry that such a system has been created in the brief period of a single century.

The reason for this explosive growth is obvious. Take this all away and life would change dramatically. Washing clothes by hand, no telephone, only candle, oil, or gas light after dark, no central heating, and travel limited to the range and whim of a horse, or the steam-train timetable. All this electrical equipment is now vital to us, and to remove it would dislocate our whole way of life, and paralyse industry. In just one century, our lives and our livelihoods have become dependent upon this new electrical and magnetic energy system.

This is a cable-based energy system. The further discovery that electricity and magnetism could be persuaded to escape from their cage of wires and spread out freely across empty space gave birth to the age of the 'wireless' as it used to be called. There is some argument about who first invented the radio – the German scientist Hertz, who is usually given the credit; or Nikola Tesla working in America; or, a complete outsider, Singh, in India, who is reported to have set off a cannon using sparks generated at a distance from the gun. All these developments took place in the 1880s.

Since this time, and growing exponentially since the late 1940s, a second and quite distinct new energy-system has been created. This comprises all the radio, TV, radar, and satellite radiation that fills the whole atmosphere of the earth and pulses around every organism on dry land. Hundreds of these kinds of transmissions are probably falling onto the surface of your eyes as you read these words, depending on exactly where you are, and which way you are facing. It is important to realise that all of these radiations are vibrating at very high frequencies.

The natural electric and magnetic oceans of the earth are therefore also changing very rapidly. Some of these changes can have a direct affect on water. Not only is water the dominant substance in living tissues, it also flows through all organisms and ecosystems. During an average human life of 70 years something like 15,000 gallons of water flow in and out of the body. A healthy mature broadleaf tree can transpire 50 gallons of water from the soil into the air in a single summer day. All organisms live in a flux of water, and in this flow the complexities of bio-chemical processes take place. From the humblest bacterium to the blue whale, all are utterly dependent upon water's diverse properties for their very existence.

Many of water's properties are very well understood, such as its ability to transport dissolved substances to and from every part of the organism, its capacity for carrying warmth, and its high surface tension – which, for example allows the formation of emulsions in milk, and colloids in cartilage formation.

However, our knowledge is far from exhaustive. Water's central role in almost every process in each and every organism, together with its electrical properties, single it out as a substance worthy of very special attention in the context of a rapidly changing electro-magnetic environment.

One key property of water that needs to be explored in this connection is its response to **vibration** and **rhythm.** These are two very basic phenomena in the present context, and we need to distinguish them clearly. Some simple examples can help clarify them for us. Let us look at three types of time-pattern, of contrasting character:

1. A simple experiment: hold your hand horizontally in front of you, level with your eyes, and keep it still for a moment or two. Think of this as a rest position. Now move your hand up and down rhythmically above and below this rest position, as if you were waving to someone... then read on.

In order to do this you had to make several decisions:

– When do I start?
– Do I move my hand up or down to begin the movement?
– How high do I lift it above the rest position?
– How far do I let my hand fall below the rest position?
– How quickly do I move my hand?
– How do I vary the speed of my hand?
– When do I stop?
– What is the 'character' of the wave?

You probably did not *think* these out one at a time, but just got on with it. However, the 'time-pattern' you made was still determined by the way in which you decided on the above questions, even if this was unconscious or semi-automatic.

In order to make this pattern more visible, take a pencil and a piece of plain paper. Put the paper on the table, and position the pencil at the lefthand side if you are right-handed. Now move your hand in the same way as you did before, but make the movement towards and away from your body, across the paper. You should now get just one straight line on the paper, over which you keep on drawing as the pencil moves. Now, keeping the rhythm of the right hand going, pull the paper sideways with your left hand at a steady rate. This should result in a line that waves up and down somewhat like **diagram 3**. To stop yourself watching what you are drawing, and therefore trying to consciously influence the pattern, it is much better to do this experiment with your eyes shut (after a bit of practice) so that you can really live into the rhythm, and then get another person to pull the paper.

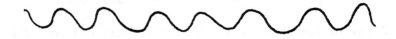

Diagram 3: Trace made by hand wave

The varieties of shape that you can draw are endless, not because you are not good enough to repeat the processes exactly, but because it is *impossible* for you to do so. A vital characteristic of natural processes is that they have *endless variations on a theme, but never repeat exactly.*

Each drawing represents a pattern of movement in time. Take **diagram 4** for example. The 'up' movement is quite slow and steady, but the down movement is so rapid that there is a 'bounce' at the bottom due to the sudden change of direction. The shape of the drawing gives a representation of the real pattern of the hand movements in time, recording them in a spatial diagram. This pattern represents the number of times your hand moved, or the *frequency* of movement.

The same, of course, happens in your handwriting every time you write a letter. It is the **form** of the trail of ink that is important, through which you communicate your sequence of thoughts. This produces a manifestation in spatial form of a time-process. The 'transformer' is the combination of your nerves, muscles, bones and other tissues, and the pen and paper. The form once drawn is more or less independent of time, but represents some characteristics of the temporal process. Such a transition from time processes to spatial forms is of particular interest in the present context of water and electromagnetism.

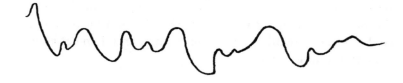

Diagram 4: Trace made by hand wave with 'bounce'

2. Let us now look at a second, somewhat less accessible example, the 13 amp electrical socket on the wall.

In the UK this has three rectangular holes. The large top hole is a safety provision, and is wired to the earth outside the house, having no direct connection with the other two holes which supply the power. The lefthand hole, the 'neutral', is always in a sort of rest position electrically, like your hand was in the above experiment, and is permanently very close to the electrical condition of the earth. The righthand hole is the dangerous one. This is the 'live' or 'line'. The electrical strength or potential of this terminal varies 'above' and 'below' that of the neutral, by a maximum of +340 volts and a minimum of - 340 volts.[4]

Between these two lower holes and in front of the socket, there is an electrical field which is oscillating all the time.

A field is a region of space which has certain definite properties. An electric field has electrical properties, while a magnetic field is a region of space having magnetic properties, and a gravitational field one in which things always move in one direction, downwards.

As electric fields go, the field round the electrical socket is not very strong, and you cannot normally sense it directly.

However, the correct instrument can enable one to make a pattern of the way in which it oscillates, which is similar to the previous diagram to the extent that it gives a spatial pattern of the way the electrical properties of the space vary over a period of time. Such a pattern looks like **diagram 5** and will be very familiar to many technical readers. The **form** of this pattern, though, *never changes* – unlike the previous one. Indeed, great efforts are made in generating electricity to see that it does not vary. This oscillating electrical field form is very close to that of a common mathematical pattern known as a 'sine' curve; it is therefore called a *sine wave,* and is of special importance in the present context.

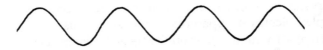

Diagram 5: Electric field at a 13 amp socket

The pattern repeats itself 50 times a second in the UK and most other countries, but 60 times a second in USA. Such repetition is known as the *frequency.* Frequency is usually measured in the number of cycles in one second, if the movement is fairly fast (cycles per second or cps, Hertz or Hz). In other words, the frequency of this mains supply electric field at the socket is 50 cycles per second, or 50 Hz. This *never changes.*

The form of this oscillating field is always a sinewave. *This also never changes.*

The strength of this field is always close to the RMS average of 240 volts, with peaks and troughs of +340 and -340 volts. *This changes very little.*

So the electric field at the socket between the two square pins has a constant frequency, a constant average strength and a constant form.

Just for clarity, the above three unvarying characteristics refer to the **electric** field at the socket, between the two lower holes. It is necessary to distinguish this from the **magnetic** field, which we will talk about later.

3. Thirdly, let us now look at a fundamental and much more complex organic rhythm: that of the heart.

A doctor or a heart specialist might wish to examine the rhythm of your heart, as this is one central indicator of your health. Out comes the stethoscope. Your heartbeat is strong enough to generate a vibration in the chest cavity, from which a trained ear can recognise a specific pattern and diagnose certain serious abnormalities. This is a pattern in time. This listening is, however, quite a crude process – although it is surprising how much a trained ear can recognise. A more complex electrical apparatus would show this pattern on the screen of a TV monitor, or on the trace drawn by a cardiograph. This is the electrocardiogram, or ECG. This machine also turns a process in time into a pattern in space.

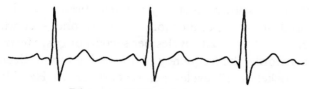

Diagram 6: Heartbeat at rest

Diagram 6 shows a typical healthy cardiogram pattern of one single heartbeat and a series of heartbeats. The single beat lasts for just under a second when you are resting. The up and down movement of the needle that traced this pattern is a reflection of the movement of the heart muscles, in the same way that the trace that you drew in the experiment (1) above was a pattern of the movement of your arm muscles. This pattern repeats around 70 times a minute in a resting state – and continues to repeat, virtually without interruption, around three billion times in a 70 year lifetime. But it is subject to many variations.

If you take the dog for a walk, win the jackpot, or go upstairs to bed, this frequency will change dramatically. The shape of this repeating pattern also changes if you begin strenuous physical work, as shown in **diagram** 7.

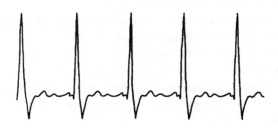

Diagram 7: Heartbeat at exercise

The frequency of the heartbeat is *never perfectly uniform,* even at rest. The expansion and contraction of the heart muscles is coupled to the breathing rate, so as you breathe in, your heart speeds up slightly, and as you breathe out it slows down. There is a constant slight variation in the rate at which the heart pulses, which is a sign of good health. Indeed, if the resting rate becomes perfectly uniform this is quite a strong indicator of impending heart disorder. The heartbeat incorporates the breathing rhythm into its own rhythm. Technically this is called a modulation. The blood pulse is modulated by the breathing rate.

The above three examples of patterns and variations in time translated into a pattern in space, demonstrate some key differences between a vibration and a rhythm. Both share three fundamental characteristics: form, frequency and strength. The key distinction between vibration and rhythm is that one has the characteristic of uniformity, whereas the other produces endless variations on a theme.

For example, strength, frequency and form of the heart-muscles' movements are subject to both dramatic and subtle variations according to the overall context of a person's physical and emotional state. The heart rhythm is representative of many other cyclical, organic processes – all organisms are an orchestrated web of myriad complex processes, each having its own pattern, and each subject to its own rhythmical changes of strength, frequency and form.

This is, of course, very close to the world of music. Volume, pitch and dynamics relate closely to strength, frequency and form. The whole world of music consists largely of endless variations of these three simple elements.

But three new players have now joined nature's orchestral music: the new electrical, electromagnetic and magnetic vibrations introduced by machines. They too have their own strengths, frequencies and patterns, but, in their new form, are not part of the orchestral score of nature. This is not simply a pleasant metaphor. The rhythms, oscillations and vibrations of nature are exquisitely orchestrated into a single whole. This is true of any organism, or any ecosystem large or small. The new patterns from electrical machines, on the other hand, are not integrated into this structure, but imposed upon it.

The orchestration, or regulation, as it is usually called in biology, of the multitude of organic processes in any organism or ecosystem, is a subject of hot debate, and intense research. Whilst an enormous amount of detail is known about individual processes, clear answers to the question of how such regulation is governed and managed remain elusive. What is clear is that both electricity and magnetism are factors which can affect many organic processes and so influence the dynamics and regulation of any system.

Pioneer research has been done in this field by people such as Robert Becker, the American surgeon, who broke quite new ground in the 1960s and 70s by uncovering a relationship between electricity and the healing of tissues after injury and surgery.[5] Professor Frohlich, for example, has demonstrated many effects of high frequency electromagnetic radiations on enzyme production.[6] In the last 25 years, a handful of other indomitable spirits have created the new scientific discipline of bioelectricity. Andrew Marino, Andrew Bassett, Zachary Friedenberg, Carl Brighton, Allen Frey, Milton Zaret, and Cyril Smith are some of the key names.[7] Work in Soviet Russia is still not easily accessible, but it is clear that competent scientists there have also discovered the physiological effects of electromagnetic fields. A number of these people have risked their careers and academic ostracism in order to establish the scientific discipline of electrobiology, which is now an accepted and respected field of research.

The overriding message from this body of research is clear: electromagnetic fields can affect biological processes.

It is also clear that

- some of these effects are harmful.
- some of these effects are not harmful
- some of these effects are healthy
- organic tissues and processes are sensitive to very low intensities of electromagnetism, particularly when it is maintained for long periods of time (i.e. 'coherent in time').
- water is central to this issue, as it is affected by electricity and magnetism.

Before going on to investigate water's vibrational properties in this context, let us first clarify a few ideas about the netherworld of electricity, magnetism and electromagnetism.

---

[1] Callahan P.S., 1977: *Tuning into Nature,* Routledge and Kegan Paul.

[2] Karl von Frisch, 1954: *The Dancing Bees,* Methuen and Co.

[3] Original German:

> *Sie rückt und weicht, der Tag ist überlebt,*
> *Dort eilt sie hin und fordert neues Leben.*
> *Oh, dass kein Flügel mich vom Boden hebt*
> *Ich nach und immer nach zu streben.*
>
> *Ein schöner Traum indessen sie entweicht.*
> *Ach, zu des Geistes Flügeln wird so leicht*
> *Kein körperlicher Flügel sich gesellen.*

[4] No, this is *not* a printing error instead of 240 volts. A mathematical sleight of hand is needed in order to get the average of these positive and negative variations, for which the simple average would be zero. You take the maximum value of + 340, and the minimum of − 340, square them, making them both positive, add them together, divide by two, square root the answer, and then divide this result by the square root of two. This gives the usual figure of 240 volts, which is an average or root mean square (RMS) value of the possible variations.

[5] Robert O. Becker and Gary Selden, 1987: *The Body Electric: Electromagnetism and the Foundations of Life,* William Morrow, New York.

[6] Frohlich and F. Kremer, 1983: *Coherent Excitations in Biological Systems,* Springer Verlag, Berlin.

[7] Cyril Smith and Simon Best, 1989: *Electromagnetic Man, Health and Hazard in the Electrical Environment,* J.M. Dent and Sons, London. Also: Andrew A. Marino (ed), 1988: Modern Bioelectricity, Marcel Dekker, New York.

Chapter 3:
Electricity, Magnetism and Electromagnetism

Though electricity and magnetism are both part and parcel of the natural environment, and both affect a very large region of space in and around the earth, they are two quite distinct forces, with different properties.

The word **field** is used as the generic term for a region of space with particular properties. An electric field is a region of space that has **electric** properties, while a magnetic field is a region of space that has **magnetic** properties. These two types of field are not mutually exclusive. It is possible to have both types of field *independently* in the same space, just as it is possible to have both sugar and salt dissolved, but chemically independent, in the same glass of water. The earth naturally has both of these fields.

Most people are completely unaware of the earth's magnetic field. As we walk, drive, eat and sleep, this field continually passes right through us – through every single blood corpuscle – but we do not experience it. However, if all the readers of this text were to be blindfolded, thoroughly disorientated by being driven to an unfamiliar environment on a dark cloudy night, and then asked to point in the direction of North, a statistically significant proportion would get it approximately correct. In other words, it seems that we *do* possess some dim awareness of the direction of the earth's magnetic field, which covers the entire surface of the earth, penetrates the oceans and all the crustal rocks, and also extends out into space far above the atmosphere in a very asymmetric form, with a long tail directed away from the sun **(diagram 8)**.

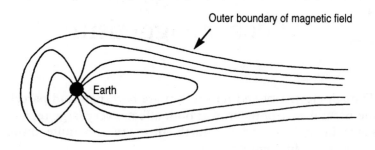

Outer boundary of magnetic field

Earth

Diagram 8: The magnetic field of the Earth

The dynamics of this field are quite complicated. The form appears to have a definite outer boundary in space, known as the 'magnetopause', which is not fixed but is influenced by a number of factors. The asymmetric form and tail are caused by radiations from the sun, which constantly stream towards the earth as it rotates on its axis in space. This axis does not coincide with the North-South axis of the magnetic field, which has its North pole in Northern Canada at present and not at the geographic North pole. This means that the magnetic field has a daily wobble as the earth rotates on its annual journey round the sun.

The earth's rotational axis in space is not vertical with respect to the plane of the earth and the sun, but is inclined at an angle of $23^{1}/2°$ to the vertical. This inclination of the axis, together with the daily rotation, creates a very complicated relative movement between the earth and the sun over the course of a year, giving rise to the seasons with all their daily and annual variations. The magnetic field of the earth is an integral part of these daily and annual changes which have their impact on its dynamics.

The moon is another very influential factor. As our nearest neighbour in space, it has a strong effect on the earth, giving rise to the ocean tides, for example. The moon is beyond the magnetopause, but, in its orbit, is constantly changing its position with respect to it as it goes through its monthly phases.

The phases of the moon – caused by its position in relation to the sun and the earth – follow a very complicated set of cycles, so that one 'moonth' is not the same length as one month. The moon takes 29 days, 12 hours, 44 minutes and 3 seconds to go through one complete cycle of phases, which is one 'moonth' or strictly one synodic or sun month. One calendar month lasts anything from 28 to 31 days depending on the time of year. One year lasts 365 days, 6 hours and 9 minutes. The moon cycle does not divide exactly into this number which means that the moon's movement does not exactly synchronise with that of the sun and therefore with the seasons. In other words you will not find the moon in the same place in the same phase on the same date in successive years.

These complicated cycles of movement are important because they all play into the dynamics of the earth's magnetic field, and all undergo patterns of change which do not quite fit into each other in a numerical sense. This gives rise to a very broad pattern of subtle change within the earth's magnetic field. The other planets also have their cycles and variations, which all influence the earth's magnetic field at a very subtle level. These interrelated movements create very complex subtle rhythms within the earth's magnetic field – and organisms are sensitive to very small levels of magnetic variation.

The strength of a magnetic field is measured in units called Teslas, named after Nikola Tesla, doyen of the world of electrical vibrations. A field with a strength of one Tesla is a very strong magnet, the strength of the earth's field being around 20,000 times weaker. One millionth of a Tesla is called a microtesla, abbreviated to 'μT'. The earth's magnetic field strength is around 40 to 7O μT, depending on location, with an average of around 5O μT. It is this weak field that orientates the compass which guided early navigators across the world's oceans.

There is an even smaller sub-division of the Tesla, which is one thousandth of one microtesla, or one thousand millionth of a Tesla; this is the nanotesla, written 'nT' for short. A field of 1 nT is a *very weak* magnetic field. The birds and the bees know a thing or two, and both appear to be able to detect magnetic fields of around this magnitude, that is *fifty thousand* times weaker than the earth's field strength, for their own basic navigation [4]. The human pineal gland is one of the key organs of regulation, which is known to have magnetic sensitivity with a theoretical lower limit of 0.24 nT, or *two hundred thousand* times weaker than the earth's magnetic field strength [4]. This may explain how people can find North, even when blindfolded. Current research is investigating organisms and magnetic field strengths that are one hundred thousand times weaker than even this weak nanotesla field.

Sensitivity to magnetic fields of this order means that some organisms are able to respond to very small levels of change in the general background level of magnetic field strength. It is clear from experimental work that both birds and bees are very finely tuned to their magnetic environment for navigation, migration and foraging.

This level of animal, insect and human magnetic sensitivity also needs to be seen in relation to our domestic and industrial electrical and magnetic apparatus. As an example, a *single* very long wire supplying just three 100 watt light bulbs (1 Amp) will produce a magnetic field with the strength of about 1 nT at at distance of 200 metres from the wire. This means that if you stand 200 metres from this wire, you, and the birds and bees around you are just about able to respond. As you move closer, the magnetic field strength will increase. Very close to the wire the magnetic field will be roughly 200,000 times stronger, or four times the earth's magnetic field strength. It is important, however, to note that this applies to a single wire, where the electric current is flowing in one direction only. In a pair of wires, as in house wiring, the current flows in opposite directions, and the magnetic effect of the currents in each wire almost cancel each other out.

Due to these and other factors, the earth's magnetic field is not perfectly steady, but undergoes both cyclical and apparently random variations of up to 2 per cent of its steady average value. This means a variation of up to 1 μT. This is a change 1000 times bigger than the minimum for a bee to notice, for example. *This is very significant.* It means that organisms can respond to variations of only one thousandth of the earth's normal steady magnetic field, and so are sensitive to its many natural fluctuations. The strength of the magnetic field vibrations that are generated close to equipment such as computers, washing machines and central heating pumps is far above this threshold of sensitivity.

The variations in the earth's field have a number of frequencies embedded within them: cycle times of 24 hours corresponding to the rotation of the earth, 29 days related to the phases of the moon, 365 days from the earth's relative annual movement to the sun, various periods related to the magnetic storms of the 11 year sunspot cycle, and many variations from the interplanetary magnetic field. The outer surface of the magnetosphere, the 'magnetopause', is a very mobile and sensitive surface, which plays a role in mediating between these subtle rhythms from our cosmic environment and the earth.

The earth's natural magnetic field is, therefore, far from simple. It carries a range of natural cycles of change that are related to many fundamental rhythms of the whole environment of the earth, both local and distant. Its rhythms penetrate the organs and tissues of all organisms without exception, which can develop the sensitivity to respond to its variations. These magnetic rhythms are a part of our natural environment, to which we and nature have adapted. Bird migration is a case in point.

There is another characteristic of magnetic fields which is particularly relevant in the present context. *They are very difficult to get rid of.* For all practical, everyday purposes, all substances are 'transparent' to magnetic fields. It is very difficult and expensive to screen an area so that it is free from either the earth's or any other magnetic field. Iron is one substance that has a strong relationship to magnetism, but a great deal of iron is needed to eliminate the earth's magnetic field from a space such as a room. **This means, in practice, that any magnetic field generated by equipment or any other means cannot be contained or screened.**

The earth also has an electric field, of whose existence few people are aware. It reaches from the ground up to the upper atmosphere, the 'ionosphere', some 100 miles up. Between these two surfaces, there is an electrical voltage of 200,000 to 300,000 volts, or about 1000 times the strength of a wall socket. This creates an electrical tension and thus an electric field. The tension is measured by taking the electrical voltages between two vertical points a metre apart; this gives a value of volts per metre. At ground level this is around 100 volts per metre, which means that between the top of your head and the ground there is a voltage of about 200 volts, fairly close to that of the mains socket, but not vibrating in a sinewave. The reason that you do not get an electric shock is that there is almost no power available from this field, and your presence changes the local situation, so you normally feel nothing.

Clouds can change this electric field strength dramatically, especially if they are of the thunder variety. The field strength can then rise by a factor of 500 times to as much as 50,000 volts per metre locally. This is now enough to make you irritable, upset your concentration, and possibly cause a headache. The electric field is subject to much wider and more violent variations than the magnetic field, due to weather conditions which are notoriously unpredictable, day/night rhythms, as well as a number of regular and irregular cycles connected with the sun, which affect the ionosphere. The breath-taking Aurora Borealis or Northern Lights in the arctic region is an example of such an interaction. The earth's electric field is also subject to natural vibrations over a range of frequencies, some of them quite low, around 1-30Hz. These were theoretically predicted in the 1950's by W.O. Schumann, and in 1962 they were discovered in America by the National Bureau of Standards. They were found, as Schumann had forecast, to be almost indistinguishable from human brain wave electrical patterns. These oscillations in the earth's electrical field are now called 'Schumann Waves', and are present all day everyday in our unseen environment. They have a pronounced peak activity at around 8Hz, but range from about 1Hz to 30Hz. The human eye oscillates at several frequencies between 8Hz and 30Hz, without which you would be unable to see any images.

The fact that these frequencies are imprinted into our body functions in such critical organs as the eye and brain shows how close the coupling is between our body functions and our environment, and in particular our electrical environment.

Unlike the magnetic field, the electric field is quite easy to screen. If you cover a box with thin kitchen foil, there will be no electric field inside it. This was discovered by Michael Faraday 150 years ago; such a protected space is still often called a Faraday Cage. This means in practice that it is possible to arrange protection from an electric field by simple thin metallic screening.

The magnetic and electric fields appear to be quite distinct from each other and have differing properties, yet they interpenetrate one another. These are two separate natural 'species' of field bound to the earth, and both are capable of varying over short or long cycles of time. Each field can, quite independently, carry different vibrations over a very wide range of frequencies – taking years for some cycles, and millionths of a second for others.

But although they are quite distinct, different entities, these two species of field are closely related – so close, in fact, that one can turn into the other, rather like a caterpillar turning into a butterfly.

The key to the transformation of electricity into magnetism, and magnetism into electricity is movement. If either one vibrates, it turns in a split second into the other, by a process that so far defies clear comprehension. This begins an alternating transformation of electricity into magnetism and then of magnetism into electricity, and so on ad infinitum. Once initiated, this process spreads out through space at the modest speed of 300,000km per second, creating a dynamic 'leap-frogging' matrix of concentric electric and magnetic fields. This kind of dynamic electric and magnetic field is called an **electromagnetic** field. Because of its capacity to continuously spread out into space, it is of a fundamentally different nature from either the electric or the magnetic fields on their own, which remain relatively local, and can be stable for quite long periods of time. In contrast, the electromagnetic field is always vibrating and spreading out into space. If it stops vibrating, it ceases to exist. The range of vibrations is vast, as we shall see below.

Such fields have always existed on the earth, accompanying every flash of lightning – one every three seconds or so somewhere on the earth, so the satellites tell us. Electromagnetic vibrations of a wide range of frequencies arise from the interaction of the ionosphere, the atmosphere, and the earth's surface with radiations that arrive from far beyond our boundaries. We experience a part of this energy as light and warmth from the sun. The processes of electricity and magnetism in the upper atmosphere are extremely complex and sensitive, interacting with the rarefied gases in this region. The current increase in ultra-violet at ground level due to changes in the ozone layer is an example of how delicately these energy transformation processes are balanced.

To summarise, there are three distinct types of field, related, but with quite different properties:
Electric fields
Electromagnetic fields
Magnetic fields

Electric fields can be static or vibrating. They are fairly local, and do not spread out in space. They are easily screened from a small space. They do not penetrate many materials or organisms, generally only having an effect on their surfaces. When they vibrate they generate electromagnetic fields.

Electromagnetic fields are always vibrating; they always spread out into space indefinitely and carry alternating electric and magnetic vibrations. They can quite easily be screened from small spaces. Their degree of penetration of materials depends on the nature of the materials and the frequency of vibration.

Magnetic fields can be static or vibrating. They are fairly local and do not spread out into space. They cannot be screened, and penetrate all materials and organisms. When they vibrate they generate electromagnetic fields.

It is important to distinguish these three invisible entities, as they have differing properties and form three distinct energy systems which have different effects on water and organic tissues. They have all existed in the natural environment for long ages, and clearly form vital functions in the living world.

Recent additions to these natural fields via our electrical technology have had the effect of increasing the intensity, range and the geographical distribution of vibrations across an enormous spectrum of frequencies in all three fields. This has resulted in the creation of local and global field modifications, of which the following are typical examples.

- strong local vibrating magnetic fields, in motors for washing machines, central heating pumps and power transformers.
- a wide spectrum of global electromagnetic radiation for radio, TV, and telephones.
- strong local vibrating electric fields around overhead power lines, TV sets and computers.

The intimate relationship between these three species of field makes it difficult to get a clear view of what is happening in any given practical situation, but luckily there is a simple rule of thumb. The key is to know how fast the fields are vibrating, i.e. their frequency. If it is low, then the electric and the magnetic fields can be thought about quite independently for all practical purposes, and the electromagnetic field ignored. If the frequency is high, then the electric and the magnetic fields can be ignored as separate entities, and the field can be thought of as just a simple electromagnetic field.

This is a slight oversimplification, but it helps to clarify a complex issue. The question is, what is a low frequency, and what is high?

This spectrum of both natural and man-made electro-magnetic radiation is shown in **diagram 9**. (This is the second type of radiating field listed above.) The range of frequencies is difficult to imagine. The piano has a range of seven octaves, and between one octave and the next the frequency of any note doubles; so between the lowest (28Hz) and the highest (3584Hz) notes on the keyboard, the frequency doubles seven times: (2^7x28=3584).

On the electromagnetic spectrum the frequency between the household mains at 50Hz and X-rays at 1,000,000,000,000,000,000Hz doubles around sixty times, the equivalent of eight piano keyboards. The total electromagnetic spectrum is around 100 octaves with no clear beginning or end. In quite a large proportion of this electromagnetic keyboard, both natural and man-made vibrations can now be found, with some frequencies more dominant than others, such as the 50Hz mains power.

There is a significant threshold in this spectrum. It took the death of some 500 scientists (the so-called X-ray martyrs) in the half century following the discoveries of radioactivity and X-rays in the 1890s, to understand that these radiations are

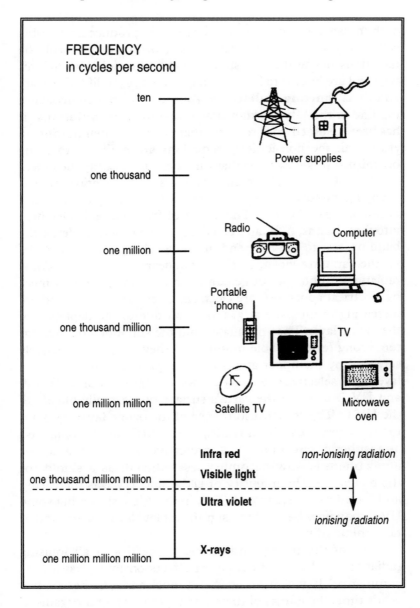

Diagram 9: The spectrum of electromagnetic radiation now present on the Earth

both mutagenic and carcinogenic; i.e. they produce irreversible cell changes and cause cancerous growth of cells. All the radiations below the line shown in the ultraviolet, are of this type and are known to be extremely dangerous to life. These are known as **ionising radiations.** All the other radiations above the line in the UV are known as **non-ionising radiations**. It has been assumed until recently, that except for their heating up effects, all the non-ionising radiations are harmless to living organisms. It is now clear that this is not necessarily the case.

The **ultra-violet** region deserves special mention, as it is changing rapidly and is the threshold between ionising and non-ionising radiations. This range of frequencies is classified into three bands, A, B, and C. UV A, the near ultra-violet, is the band nearest to the blue end of the visible spectrum, and UV C, the far ultra-violet, is the band nearest to X-rays. These radiations, although not generated in the general environment by electrical apparatus, are electromagnetic radiations, and are increasing in intensity at ground level due to the depletion of the ozone layer. They originate from the sun, but would be far too strong for the whole biosphere if they were not selectively screened by the upper atmosphere, in particular by the ozone layer. The selective screening allows a proportion of the UV A and UV B to reach the earth's surface but virtually blocks all the UV C. The recent disturbance of the ozone layer by man-made chemicals is affecting this delicately balanced atmospheric screening. The protective skin of the upper atmosphere is now becoming less efficient as a shield for the biosphere. The intensity of UV A and UV B is increasing and recent measurements (1994), in the Alps, show that some UV C may now be reaching significant levels on the ground at fairly high altitude.

One of the poorly understood properties of all ionising radiations is that their damaging effects on living tissues are cumulative. If you have an X-ray now and another in two year's time, the effects of these add together in your organism. All your exposure to such radiations adds up in your life. There is now some evidence that this also may apply for some of the non-ionising radiations as well, right down to frequencies of 50/60Hz.

A distinction was made above between high and low frequencies in relation to electric and magnetic fields. This is not a distinction with the same clarity as that between ionising and non-ionising radiations, and is much more of a convenience or rule of thumb.

The most common low-frequency equipment is everything connected to the main electrical power supply at 50 or 60 Hz. At this frequency the electric field and the magnetic field can be considered as quite distinct fields, and the electromagnetic field is irrelevant. As the frequency of a system goes up the situation slowly reverses; and so, at the medium waveband BBC broadcast frequency, which is around 1 million Hz, the electromagnetic field is important and the electric and magnetic fields can be ignored. So, in all issues connected with mains electricity, the electric and magnetic fields need to be considered independently from each other, and for all radio, TV, satellite and portable phone transmissions only the effects of the electromagnetic field are relevant and the electric and magnetic fields can be ignored.

The electric, magnetic and electromagnetic fields, both natural and man-made, are three closely related energy systems. They are all in a state of vibration due to many factors. We therefore live in a vibrating matrix of electricity and magnetism, part of it natural and part of it man-made. The natural background vibrations carry constantly changing modulations or rhythms originating from the manifold aspects of natural processes. The man-made vibrations act in the same medium, but do not carry the same naturally ordered, modulating rhythms.

The phenomenon of man-made, electromagnetic 'noise' or interference has infiltrated the 'silence' of the natural electromagnetic world.

This noise is not uniformly distributed, but on the contrary, shows enormous variation from one situation to another. The trouble is that we cannot hear it with our ears, or perceive it directly through any of our senses – but it exists as a disturbance which affects the whole biosphere, of which water is such an integral and vital part.

Chapter 4:
Water as a Carrier of Information Patterns

Heart-stimulant drugs can increase the rate at which the heart beats. Distilled water, or just pure water, has no such stimulant effect on the heart – or so it was thought before Benveniste[1] and his colleagues got to work in Paris.

They took a standard stimulant drug dissolved in distilled water and applied it to the heart of a rat, causing a dramatic increase in its pulse-rate. Then they repeated the experiment, but used only distilled water with nothing dissolved in it. This had no effect whatsoever. They then 'imprinted' the drug onto a similar sample of distilled water with nothing dissolved in it, through a special electromagnetic process, after which the water was *still* only distilled water with nothing dissolved in it. But when this was applied to the rat's heart, the pulse-rate again increased dramatically. *They had managed to transfer some property of the drug to the water without using any of its physical substance.* This very remarkable experiment was shown in detail on a BBC documentary series 'Heretic' [2] in 1994. The experiment was ridiculed as being impossible and caused a furore in some sections of the scientific community. It appears from this that 'pure' water is a very interesting substance.

Rainwater, tapwater, ditchwater, polluted water, holy water, distilled water, pondwater, sweet water, black water, grey water, brackish water, salt water, spa water, hard water, soft water, and of course pure fresh bubbling healthy spring water. There are many types of water, but what distinguishes one from another?

The general and much publicised pollution of water supplies is beginning to wake us up to what water contains, as we think twice about drinking a cocktail of nasties, however dilute: so the sales of bottled water soar. This is 'pure spring water', and therefore, by definition, healthy to drink. But is it pure and 'healthy', and what makes spring water so attractive?

Water is capable of dissolving a very large range of substances, more than any other liquid. The saturation level – the point at which no more substance will dissolve – is quite high for salt. Limestone dissolves in water too, as those living in hard water areas know only too well, but the saturation level is quite low. Iron, in the form of rust, also dissolves in water, but the saturation level is very low. Many minerals are slightly soluble in water, and form its natural content as it emerges from the ground. The range and concentration of these minerals depend on the geological strata that the water has passed through, and how long it dwelt there. Each natural spring has a different spectrum of minerals in it, with widely varying concentrations. Some will be at the saturation level, others only present in trace quantities. This is a factor which distinguishes one source of water from another.

Rain water originates in nature's still, from the surface of the oceans and rivers, and from the immeasurably large area of plant leaves on the earth. It evaporates from these sources as water with no dissolved minerals, but as it begins to condense, it picks up oxygen, nitrogen and carbon dioxide at quite low levels of concentration, since these gases are slightly soluble in water.

Soluble and insoluble elements soon join the gases as the water forms, travels as clouds, and then falls to the ground with an abundant harvest of suspended and dissolved substances. Some of these come from natural sources such as dust, salt from ocean spray, pollen grains, and bacteria. Oxides of nitrogen and sulphur, and agricultural chemicals, on the other hand, come from industry. As each drop falls, it travels through the magnetic, the electric and the electromagnetic fields of the earth.

The substance-pollution of water that has become so widespread is due to one of three basic causes:

- dissolved or suspended substances that are directly harmful, such as dust, pesticides or industrial waste (for example, acid rain, smog, and agricultural run-off water).
- an excess of substances normally found in water, such as nitrates or organic waste (typically sewage).
- harmful micro-organisms, and infectious bacteria (such as salmonella germs).

Pure water, from a technical point of view, contains nothing but water, obtained by distillation, which separates the water from all the dissolved and suspended substances listed above, except the gases. Water of such chemical purity does not occur naturally. Such water is both chemically and bacteriologically sterile, and cannot normally be found in the natural environment.

'Pure' spring water is certainly not pure in this chemical sense. Dissolved trace minerals, gathered during its long subterranean wanderings, sent crowds flocking 'to take the waters' a hundred years ago in spa towns across Europe. One thing that we hope it does not contain is any of the 100,000 or so new, man-made substances that have found their way into the surface waters of the planet in the last century. This may or may not be a well-founded hope, depending on the source of the water. If the spring is fed solely from a very deep source rising to the surface, then the water may not have seen the light of day for centuries, and may therefore be uncontaminated. Deep bore-hole water, pumped to the surface may similarly have escaped contamination, effectively having been in storage in the earth for centuries or even millenia. In some rare cases, such as certain small springs in south-west Wales, the water may never have been part of the hydrological cycle on the surface and in the atmosphere; it is called 'juvenile' water for this reason, and can possess unusual properties.

Water that emerges from the ground is not simply water. It can have a whole range of properties depending upon its recent and more ancient biography.

Its history will determine what substances it contains, and in what proportions. River water, for example, may be extracted, purified, used and returned to the river in the waste stream several times before it reaches the sea. Something tells us that this is probably acceptable for washing clothes, but not for making cups of tea. The idea of drinking someone else's waste water is not very attractive. Such recycled water can easily find its way back into the ground water through swallow holes in the bed of the river, which are springs in reverse: water disappears down the hole like a drain into the depths of the earth. Such holes are common where there are limestone or chalk outcrops in the riverbed, and mean that contaminated surface water can enter the groundwater before it is extracted for use as 'pure' mineral water.

Surely, the very real attraction of bubbling fresh spring water is not only its bounty of dissolved minerals, and the hopeful lack of contamination, but also that little extra *je ne sais quoi* that gives it vitality? What is this little extra? Is it just a romantic dream, or is there something real behind it? Are all the accounts of healing at holy springs just part of folklore, or can water carry unusual properties at certain places on the earth, such as Lourdes? If you have a good palate you can tell the difference between good quality water and tap water. You can have a sense for its quality. So do animals; they can be very selective about the water they drink, both in the wild and, given the choice, domestically.

Water has been described by one leading expert as probably the most researched and least understood liquid on the planet, as it has so many unusual and anomalous properties.[3] For example, as hot water cools from 100°C to 4°C it contracts, as do almost all other substances. But as it cools from 4°C to 0°C it expands, unlike any other substance except for the molten metal antimony. The popular view is that when the temperature of water reaches 0°C it freezes, but this is not so for pure water. Water that is chemically quite pure, and contains no particles of suspended substance, does not start to freeze until its temperature falls below 0°C by several degrees; this is known as supercooling. At a certain sub-zero temperature, depending on a number of conditions, it will quite suddenly begin to turn into solid ice, whereupon its temperature quickly rises back to zero. Pure water in very fine capillary tubes can be cooled down to -39°C and still remain a liquid. Such supercooling is one way in which some plant tissues are thought to resist freezing at sub-zero temperatures.

Recent research in Israel has also shown that a very thin layer of water held between two flat plates, suddenly behaves as if it were a solid at a critical thickness. At seven molecules thick it is a liquid, but at six molecules thick it becomes a solid.

Such examples demonstrate water's very unusual behaviour.

The above considerations are connected with the physical substances that water carries. Only pure water remains if they are all removed, but in practice this is very difficult to achieve, as even some of the glass or plastic container will dissolve to some extent in distilled water. Most of the following discussion, though, is concerned only with pure distilled water that is considered to have no dissolved substances in it apart from air-gases. This is important, as we have to consider other aspects of water's content, which are *not* of the nature of physical substance.

Everyone recognizes the formula H_2O as a chemical symbol for water. This originally derived from the practical laboratory experiment which grew out of the discovery that electricity has effects upon chemistry. In this experiment, electricity was passed through water, producing the two gases oxygen and hydrogen. This was first done last century, and is now a standard school lab experiment. **(diagram 10)**. The volumes of the two gases are produced in the ratio of 2:1 – in other words twice as much hydrogen as oxygen. The conclusion drawn from this experiment, which led to the H_2O formula, is that twice as much hydrogen as oxygen exists in water.

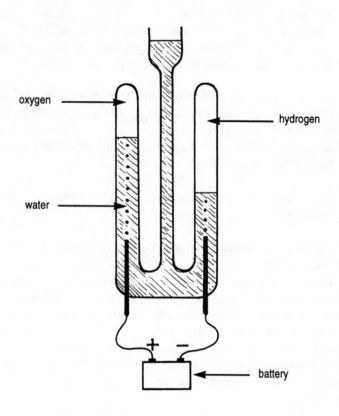

oxygen

hydrogen

water

battery

Diagram 10: Electrolysis of water. Hydrogen and oxygen are produced in the ratio of 2:1

The further conceptual elaboration of this result has led to the *theory* that water is composed of two atoms of hydrogen and one of oxygen. The formula is therefore also taken to represent the number of atoms in a molecule. The molecule of water is considered to be the smallest particle of water that can retain water's properties. The atoms are thought to be the component parts of the molecule. This atomic model of water is usually given a structural form, as shown in **diagram 11**. It has electrical charges at both ends.

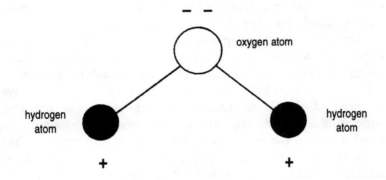

Diagram 11: Conventional atomic model of the water molecule

This picture of the molecular structure of water presents a problem in relation to the more subtle properties of water. The experiment described at the beginning of this chapter, together with the examples given in Chapter 6 show unequivocally that water even in its pure state is capable of altering biological process. This is an established practical fact. This means that pure water is able to accommodate certain information within its structure that is relevant to biological processes. The molecular model described above is not able to accommodate this experimental fact. This is why these phenomena are usually ignored by conventional scientific thinking.

This presents a dilemma. Either the facts are wrong or the molecular model is wrong or there is another aspect of water to be taken into consideration. Both the facts and the model are well established, which means that there is another dimension to the structure of water that accounts for the experimental evidence.

It seems that water molecules are able to join together and form three dimensional structures comprising a number of molecules. These form in such a way that they create a sort of shell or cage with a space inside technically known as a clathrate. These are known as the microstructures of water. Under certain conditions it is possible for other molecules to be trapped inside the cage of the microstructures.

One interesting example of such a phenomenon was found some years ago, like sunken treasure, on the floor of the Arctic Ocean. Because water is most dense and therefore smallest at 4°C, it sinks to the bottom at this temperature, which is the case in parts of the Arctic Ocean. On the bottom of the sea, depending on the depth, water is under considerable pressure. Cold water on the ocean floor, under quite high pressure has absorbed very large quantities of methane gas into its microstructure, and formed a material that somewhat resembles ice. This quasi-solid substance covers quite large areas of the Arctic Ocean floor, and is a potential source of methane gas. If it is simply brought to the surface, then it 'fizzes' as the pressure drops, releasing gaseous methane, and the solid structure disintegrates to liquid water. Such a material is an extreme example of a water clathrate in which myriads of water microstructure 'cages' hold large quantities of other molecules – in this case, methane – and form a new type of material.

Such a picture of a cluster of molecules presents a very different picture to that of the simple atomic model. This already far from simple picture is further complicated by an additional factor.

The two substances involved in forming these microstructures come in more than one form in nature. Oxygen and hydrogen, can each be found as several types, called isotopes.

These are the identical twins and triplets of the chemical world; they look the same on the outside, but are different on the inside. Oxygen can be found in three stable isotope forms. These are known as oxygen 16, 17 and 18. If you were to take a jar of pure oxygen extracted from the air, it would contain 99.76% oxygen type 16, 0.038% oxygen type 17, and 0.202% oxygen type 18.

These three different substances have identical chemical properties, but have different physical properties. Type 18 would be heavier than type 16, for example. The same goes for hydrogen, which has two stable isotopes, hydrogen 1 and hydrogen 2. Water made from hydrogen 2 is heavier than water made from hydrogen 1. This creates two types of water, one physically heavier than the other, known as heavy water. This is never found in isolation in nature, but a very small proportion is contained in every glass of water you drink. The operation of separating the two types of water is extremely difficult, and needs very large industrial equipment.

Processes in the upper atmosphere and also in the radioactive depths of the earth can create a third, unstable type of hydrogen, known as hydrogen 3, which is radioactive. (Its radioactivity halves in 12.3 years.) This occurs in nature, and is constantly breaking down and being regenerated.

All these subtly different varieties of the constituent vibrations of hydrogen and oxygen, when incorporated into water molecules give another level of complication of these structures, even if some of these elements are rare.

These microstructures are a key to understanding important aspects of water's role in living organisms.

If you strike a bell, it starts vibrating, generating a sound whose pitch and quality depend entirely on the bell's physical size and properties, how and where it is hit, and the material of the striker. The vibrations and sound will last for about 30 seconds or so, and fade away to nothing. One almost universal feature of the mechanical world is that things run down, wear out and fade away.

In complete contrast, one of the apparent anomalies of the molecular world is that it is in continuous vibration – things never run down, do not wear out and **vibrations never fade away.** At the molecular level, everything is a sea of highly organised, perpetually spinning vibrations of energy.

The clathrate microstructures are capable of vibrating as a complete entity, similar to a bell, but with one outstanding difference; no vibration that is established in the microstructure ever fades with time. Each type of microstructure can resonate to, and maintain not just one but a range of vibrational patterns.

The vibrations in a bell that is struck cause a quite complicated change in the bell's subtle shape. Some parts move outwards, while others, at the same instant, move inwards, rather like a three dimensional see-saw. This is impossible to see with the unaided naked eye. But it is possible to make a similar phenomenon visible if you look carefully: there is an after dinner party trick with an empty wine glass. If you moisten your finger, press it on the rim, and rotate it slowly round the glass, you can set the glass vibrating so that it emits a high-pitched tone **(diagram 12)**. The pitch of the tone will depend on the physical characteristics of the glass. If you now put a small quantity of water in the glass, so that it is $1/4$ to $1/2$ full, and repeat the experiment, you can see small regions of vibration on the water surface close to the glass, that travel round at the same rate as your finger, but at several fixed points relative to each other. These points are caused by the vibration of the glass, which is moving at different rates in different places, forming a pattern. We do not usually think of glass as being flexible, but in this instance, the glass is bending in and out at a few thousand times a second, and the glass adopts a particular dynamic form related to the sound.

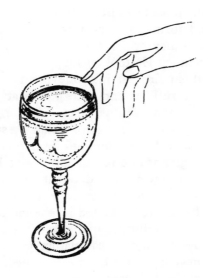

Diagram 12: Glass being vibrated with a finger

High speed photographs of the front plate of a violin taken while it is being played, show that the wood moves in a very beautiful pattern over the surface, the shape of which depends on the notes and chords being played. Movement caused by vibration can form complex patterns in space. This is another example of transitions between processes in time, and spatial form. Vibration can generate forms, provided that the receiving substances are tuned to the vibration. If you try to force the bell to vibrate at a frequency that it does not naturally adopt, it will make no sound, and the spatial movement and form will not develop.

Every object has its own particular set of frequencies to which it will naturally respond by vibrating. This is the mechanical principle of all musical instruments. The tension of a string, the length of a string, the length of a column of air are all adjusted to be tuned to one particualr frequency and its associated harmonics. Each time it is made to vibrate, it adopts some specific oscillating shape to which the vibrations are midwife.

One of the most beautiful examples of the relation between vibration and form was discovered by Friedrich Chladni, a pioneer experimenter in sound in Germany in the late eighteenth century. He took metal plates of various shapes and sizes, held them firm at just one point, spread a very fine powder on the surface, and then played at one edge of them with a violin bow, setting them vibrating. The result so impressed Napoleon that he gave Chladni a substantial grant to translate his book *Die Akustik* into French in 1802.

The photographs in **photograph 1** are taken of such a plate before and after bowing. The different patterns arise by bowing at different points round the edge of the plate. The quite unexpected forms are generated by the vibrating movement of the plate under the influence of the bow. The same piece of metal has many ways in which it can naturally vibrate, but once one pattern of movement has been established, this becomes the dominant form and all others are suppressed by the strength of this one pattern of movement. This is a clear example of how vibration, a process in time, can be transformed into a pattern in space. Once established, the pattern can persist for an indefinite time, even when the movement of the plate has long since ceased.

These examples all show how time processes become patterns in space, which are more or less independent of time, but nevertheless bear within them an image of the original pattern of movement. The same process was explored in Chapter 2 with the hand and heart rhythms

Any pattern is a source of information. We live in a world awash with information, but what is it? If you set about cooking a simple supper and clearing up afterwards in your own home, you can do it more or less automatically because you know where everything lives in the kitchen. But if you go to a friend's house to do the same thing, you will need to be told or to find out where everything is and how everything works in order to do the same job that you did at home. Once you have been initiated into the idiosyncrasies of your friend's gas-stove and kitchen drawers, you can rapidly establish a new pattern of cooking behaviour that fits the new kitchen.

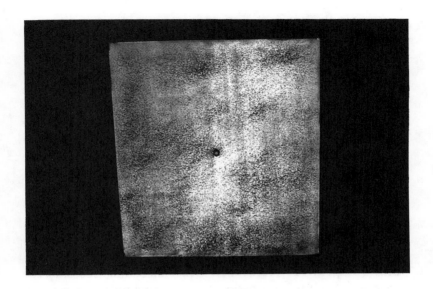

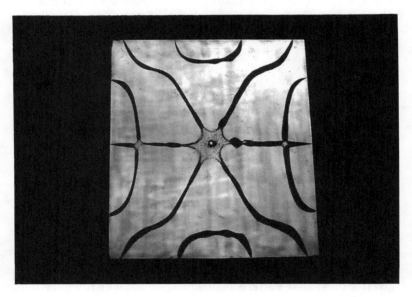

Photograph 1: A metal plate: (top) before bowing and (below) after bowing, showing vibration patterns

So information tells us about the relationship between things: this is here, that is there, there is no milk in the fridge, and so on. From a set or pattern of relationships, patterns of activity can be created. This is the reverse process from the one we have been examining, in which time processes generate spatial patterns. Information is only of any value if at some point in time it can be used to order new activity. Railway timetables are packed with information, but this is only of any value if people take them as the basis for their rail-travel. The **pattern of information orders future activity.**

Such patterns have become very common in the last couple of decades, with the rapid expansion of electronic equipment. Most products in the supermarket carry a bar code which consists of a series of upright black lines on a light background. The pattern is totally meaningless without a machine to activate it (**diagram 13**). Activation means that something starts to move and then the information code can ring up a charge at the check-out and alter the stock control level of that particular item on the company's records. The information pattern of the bar code can set off a series of meaningful actions.

Diagram 13: Bar-code information pattern of black and white stripes

Most people now use a credit or charge card of some sort for financial transactions. The card has a brown stripe on it which is a patch of paint with magnetic properties (**diagram 14**). It is given a particular pattern of magnetism for which we have no sense, but which can be 'read' by a cash point machine, for instance. The spatial magnetic pattern allows access when brought into movement by the machine. The hole in the wall hands out money at your request when activated by a magnetic pattern.

These are examples of fairly simple information patterns translating a pattern in space into an ordered activity in time, which is the key function of any information pattern.

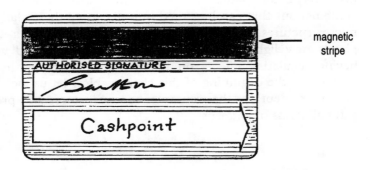

Diagram 14: Credit card information pattern of magnetism

Returning to the microstructures in water, it appears that these minute forms are able to act in a similar way as carriers of information. They can be set into vibrating patterns which have relevance for organic processes. The vibrating patterns can have an indefinite life, as explained previously, and so can hold patterns with the potential to order future activity in the organism.

This perspective throws a totally new light on the role of water in living organisms. Not only does it act as a carrier of dissolved subtances and warmth, but it also carries a library of *information* for the organic world. This information is its *vibrational* as distinct from its *material* content.

Spring water is usually rich in such patterns. This is the *je ne sais quoi*, the little extra that draws people to drink fresh spring water, and take the healing waters of the holy springs over the centuries. This is what leads animals to select one source of water rather than another. Water can be as full of vibrating information patterns as a book is full of printed information patterns on every page.

Water can contain physical substances *and* vibrational information patterns. *Both* are vital for the health of all organisms.

The microstructure of water is a storage medium for vibrating information patterns. The possible range of vibrational combinations that can be stored in water using these clathrate microstructures is immense. This perspective throws a completely new light on the apparent enigma of distilled water having regulating effects on biological processes, as in the example at the beginning of this chapter. Now let us look in a little more depth at the way water receives, stores and propagates all kinds of patterns.

---

[1] Davenas E. Benveniste J. et al., 1988: 'Human basophil degranulation triggered by very dilute antiserum against IgE' in *Nature,* vol. 333, p.816.

[2] Benveniste J., 1994: 'Heretic', a BBC 2 documentary shown on 6/2/94.

[3] Felix, Franks (ed), 1972: *A Comprehensive Treatise on Water.* 7 vols. Plenum Press, New York.

Chapter 5:
Water as a Musical Instrument

The information patterns in the water microstructure are patterns of vibration, just as a chord of five notes played on the piano is a pattern of vibrations.

The sound vibrations of chords have a very definite effect upon us, depending on the **ratios** of the frequencies. A concert-pitch piano has its A above middle C tuned to 440Hz. The middle C then has a frequency of 264Hz. One third above this, E vibrates at 330Hz and the F one semi-tone above that at 352Hz (all on the diatonic, untempered scale). The interval of the semi-tone between E and F has a frequency difference of 22 cycles a second. It is possible for a singer with a well-trained ear to distinguish up to *twelve* different tones within this one semi-tone interval. This means that at around this pitch the singer can hear the difference of about two cycles a second, a variation of only 0.6% in the frequency, or 6 parts in a thousand. So finely tuned is human sensitivity to sound!

You do not, of course, hear frequencies, but tone and *ratios* of tones generated by frequency patterns in your ear. A major third is a major third wherever it is played on the keyboard, but the frequencies must be in the ratio of $1:1\frac{1}{4}$.

The question of ratios is all important. When an orchestra plays a complex chord, there are a multitude of frequencies if all the instruments and their individual harmonics are taken into account. If just one instrument plays a wrong note, then the whole musical expression becomes discordant for us through our experience of the disturbance in the *ratio pattern* of the frequencies.

It is vital, then, that every frequency is correct *in proportion to all the others;* if it is not, then everything is affected. This is elementary in the world of music, which so obviously connects with the spectrum of audio frequencies in the air. Organisms respond to many other levels of vibration, and the principle of harmonic ratios and patterns seems to be a universal principle in living processes. The pioneer work of Tomatis in Paris has shown how sound and patterns of sound can have a dramatic healing effect on people suffering from serious chronic disorders[1]. Vibrating patterns are very powerful in organic processes. When they are correctly tuned to the organism's need, they can harmonize and heal; if they are discordant, they can cause harm.

Water is a carrier of vibrating patterns, which are patterns of information that can be of use to an organism. The patterns contain many frequencies in a particular proportion to one another. The pattern is a pattern of proportion or ratios held stable in the microstructure. Such structures are physically very small, quite specifically ordered, with patterns of immense variety. The primary source of these patterns is physical substance.

As we have seen, water is a wonderful solvent. All organic tissues are formed through the agency of substances dissolved in water. One of the most extraordinary features of organic tissues is that they are continually poised on the edge of being dissolved by the body's fluids. Everything we eat is either dissolved in the juices of the digestive tract or excreted as an indigestible solid. When any substance dissolves in water it comes into very intimate connection with the water microstructures.

Every chemical element has its own unique vibratory pattern, whether it is dissolved in water or not.

One form of this can be observed by means of an instrument called a spectroscope, which passes light through a substance in gaseous form, giving rise to a coloured spectrum consisting of a number of closely packed coloured lines. This is just a very sophisticated modification of the brilliant rainbow effect created by early autumn morning sunlight on a fresh dew drop, viewed at just the right angle. These lines form a pattern that is only created by that substance, rather like the bar code on a packet of sugar. This coloured spectrum is the unique 'signature' of the substance vibrating in a pattern of light frequencies. Our rather bilious, yellow street-lights, for example, are filled with the vapour of the metal sodium, which vibrates at just two specific frequencies in the yellow part of the spectrum. These two frequencies are unique to sodium, so they always indicates sodium's presence.

This vibrating pattern property of substance is widely used in the detection of traces of substance – in water-quality testing, for example. Silver can be detected by this means at concentrations as low as one part of silver in one million, million parts of water. In this process, a specific set or pattern of frequencies is detected and recognised, which can only be found in the physical presence of silver.

Substances have a unique vibrating pattern, 'bar code' or chord, which has a set of specific proportions. The optical process described above is just one way in which such vibrating properties can be recognised.

The proportions or ratios of the substance's vibration patterns can be transferred to vibrating patterns of the clathrate microstructures of water, provided that

- the appropriate structures are available, and
- there is an appropriate process of transfer.

The frequencies of the two media may not be the same, but the *ratios* of the frequencies, or their mutual proportions, can be preserved in a *different* vibrating medium. The 'music' is preserved, but transposed to a different octave in a different medium.

We actually use this process every day, whenever we use the telephone **(diagram 15)**. Our voice creates a specific pattern of vibrations in the air, which consists of a set of frequencies over a given period of time. These enter a microphone, hit a tiny sheet of thin metal, and set it vibrating mechanically. Here a transfer takes place of a vibrating pattern of frequencies from one medium, air, to another, metal. The metal then sets a small magnet vibrating, which in turn starts electricity in the wires vibrating. Here are two further transfers of the vibration pattern into magnetism and electricity. All that is left of the original sound vibrations in the air is the frequency pattern; everything else has changed. Air and electricity are totally different media, with very different properties. The properties of electricity can now be used to send this vibrating pattern to almost any point on the earth in a fraction of a second, using radio frequency vibrations at a much higher frequency, but with the same proportional variations. At the receiving end, the whole process can be reversed and electrical vibrations transferred back into air vibrations. The process is one of exquisitely engineered frequency management.

If at any stage in the transfer process some of the frequencies are lost, altered, or any new ones are added, the integrity of the whole pattern is compromised, leading to a distortion of the original. The voice then sounds different, or is unintelligible, at the receiving end. 'Hi-fi' stands for 'High Fidelity' or *faithful* sound reproduction. Great efforts have been made by the design engineers of such equipment, so that the vibrational patterns from the original studio sounds, through a number of transfer processes, are faithfully preserved and reproduced in the vibrations of the air in the room where you are listening. That is what you pay for in your Hi-fi: integrity in the transfer process of frequency patterns.

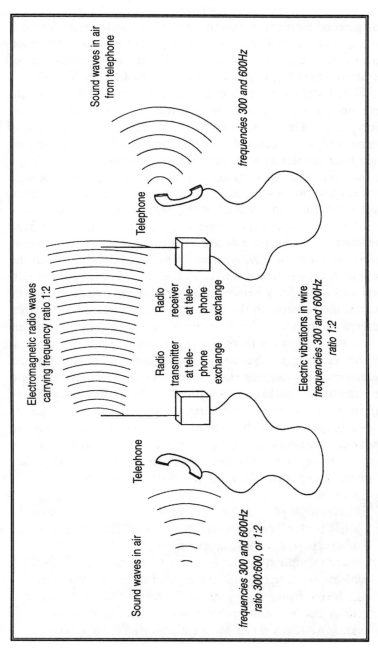

Diagram 15: Transfer of frequency proportions through the telephone system

An essential element in this process of frequency transfer from one medium to another is that there must be something which 'speaks' the language of each medium, as the transfer of vibrations takes place from one medium to another. The air and the electricity, in the above example of the telephone, would have no connection with each other if it were not for the microphone. This instrument 'speaks' both the languages of mechanical, and electrical vibration, and can bring the two into a working relationship. It acts as the go-between, so that the frequencies can have clear, unobstructed right of passage between the two media, air and electricity. The same is true in reverse for the loud speaker, or the earpiece of the telephone.

In the case of the telephone, the transfer of vibrations from one medium to another is almost instantaneous, and conversation can take place without any significant delay between the spoken and the received words. In the case of Hi-Fi equipment, there is a long delay between the air vibrations created by the musical instruments in the studio and the regenerated vibration patterns in the air of the room in which you are listening. This is, of course, because there is a recording stage in the process. In the recording, the vibration sequences in the air are transformed into a magnetic pattern on the recording tape, and are effectively 'parked' there indefinitely, simply as areas of differing strengths of magnetism. The original sequence of vibrations created by the singer's voice, which is a process in time, has now become a magnetic pattern on the tape, a pattern in space. Reversing the recording process re-creates a sequence of vibrations in time, allowing the music to be heard

This transfer of a time-based vibrational process into a spatial pattern and vice versa is central to so much of our media technology: tapes, videos, CDs. The CD disc consists simply of a circular sheet of aluminium covered with millions upon millions of tiny dents, all identical, but formed into a very precise pattern. Only when the disc is put into movement can the pattern of dents be recreated into a series of vibrations, which are a faithful reproduction of the vibrations that were originally transferred to the medium of the disc in the studio. Again, the dents are an information pattern.

In these familiar examples, then, there are two distinct processes. The first is to transfer vibrational sequences from one medium to another, with virtually no time delay; this process requires the microphone as a 'go-between'. The second is to transform a set of transient vibrations into a pattern so that it is 'recorded'; this process requires magnetic patterns on tape or dents in aluminium as a 'parking' or information medium.

The microstructure of water appears to act in a similar way. First it acts as a go-between for the frequency patterns originating from different media. Secondly, it also acts as a recording medium for vibration patterns.

In any organism there is a confluence of three distinct groups of rhythms or patterns in time. One group is formed by the electromagnetic vibrations, the second group by the vibrations belonging to physical substances, and the third group by the rhythms of the life forces. Water acts as the 'medium' between frequency patterns of each of these and the whole organism.

The earliest recorded example of a transfer of vibrating patterns from substance to water was achieved by Hahnemann, who originated the medical practice of homeopathy, which made him very unpopular with his contemporaries[2]. As one element of this new practice he found a technique for imprinting the vibrations of any given substance into water. The process is absurdly simple, but demonstrates a principle: distilled water and a small quantity of a substance are shaken together. A sample is then taken from this mixture and diluted with more distilled water and shaken again. After a number of repetitions, there is no material substance left, but the water can have differing effects on organic processes, depending on the nature of the original substance in the water.

If the tissues of the moss Lycopodium are prepared in this way, and a small quantity of the resulting water is drunk, then quite definite organic reactions appear.[3] The eyes start to water, a slight headache develops, and bedrest is needed for at least 24 hours.

The apparent contradiction of *chemically pure* distilled water having an effect on living processes as a result of its dynamic history, is resolved as soon as it is recognised that it is possible to imprint the unique vibrating pattern characteristic of each substance into the microstructure of water. It is the vibrating pattern that mediates the organic effect.

When water is shaken it becomes very turbulent and tiny vortices spin at very high velocity. *This spinning form is the equivalent of the microphone*; it speaks more than one language, and can therefore transfer frequency patterns from substance to microstructures. Once the pattern of the substance is in the microstructure, the physical substance can be removed, leaving only its vibrational 'footprint' in the water. By this simple process, substance and its vibrational signature can be separated.

The life forces – unseen, but nevertheless real and vital – need the myriad variations of microstructure vibrations in an organism in order to directly influence living processes. This happens through a process of resonance with the forms of the tissues in which the water is held. The surfaces of the tissues are set into a very subtle pattern of vibration which catalyses certain specific processes in the organ. Hence a communication channel is established between the life force vibrations and the biochemical processes in the tissues.

If the microstructures, or the patterns in them, are damaged or destroyed, then the life forces cannot gain clear access to the organs. The 'medium' cannot mediate because it cannot resonate in the correct pattern. In such a situation, a specific process such as the production of an enzyme or hormone may be inhibited, promoted or totally blocked. It is like a telephone conversation with noise on the line; you cannot hear the person at the other end, and so do not know what s/he is trying to tell you to do.

Random electromagnetism seems to affect the vibrating patterns of water by interfering with the life

rhythms, modifying the resonant responses of the micro-structure elements.

In an earlier chapter we looked at the three key aspects of oscillation, frequency, strength and form. The regularity of frequency and form of the sinecurve of the 50Hz mains, contrasts strongly with the continually varying frequency, strength and form of the heart's time-patterns. The sinecurve is very rare in nature. It is difficult to find any organic process that consistently shows such a constant pattern of variation in time. One of the key features of organic rhythms is, as we have seen, that all three oscillation characteristics **constantly vary**. In other words there are rhythms within rhythms within rhythms, embedded in each other just like the organic tissues themselves, which form a series of surfaces nesting one inside the other. These two are complementary aspects – the nesting of form within form in space, and the nesting of rhythm within rhythm in time.

The embedded rhythms and the nesting forms are intimately related, as can be seen on almost any sea shell, where the deposition of calcium carbonate from the living tissues forms varying patterns on the shell surface. The concentric rings in the trunk of deciduous trees are another example. Here the annual cycle of the year is imprinted into the form. On elm wood, it is possible to see finer rings within the strong annual ring, which reflect the moon's monthly cycle.

The sinewave, referred to in Chapter 2, is fundamental to the nature of the electrical world of power and communications. Through the electric and magnetic fields, this form in time, with its consistent frequency and form, is now superimposed on the nested matrix of organic rhythms. This can generate the 'dripping tap torture' syndrome. If you are exposed to a regular sound that repeats and repeats without variation or end it can drive you mad. Boredom and life are mutually exclusive. Endless, unaltering repetition is one of the characteristics of electrical processes. Endless variations on a theme is one of the characteristics of the organic world.

Chronic exposure to such regular background vibration can consistently damage certain specific information patterns, which have then to be constantly rebuilt by the organism. The conflict between unending regularity of electromagnetic fields and the life rhythms' continual flux, can give rise to stress. Many areas of research into the effects of electromagnetic vibrations indicate that long exposure to very low levels of disturbance can be far more harmful than higher intensity for shorter times. This introduces the concept of coherence, the term used for a vibration that is locked onto one frequency for a very long time. Coherent electromagnetic oscillations at low levels are now under close scrutiny, as this is the type of exposure that many people now have to mains and radio vibrations.

What has been outlined in this chapter is a key to understanding the way in which electricity affects us and other organisms. Water has two doorways; one into the world of electromagnetism, and one into the world of life. Both doorways lead to the vibrating inner microstructure. A harmonious confluence of these two very different worlds leads to health. A discordant confluence leads to illness.

The new, 'noisy' electromagnetic environment can modify the vibrational patterns in water in many ways, and the resulting change can bring about a variety of modifications to the way in which life processes can act in any particular organic function. Damage to the vibrational pattern of a complex microstructure may weaken an organic process. Total chaotisation of the patterns through random electromagnetic noise can seriously inhibit or block a process. Selective reinforcement of particular frequency combinations in the water-pattern may enhance the activity of a particular process. This latter case is probably an important factor in the observed phenomenon of synergy between certain particular electromagnetic frequencies and certain toxins in the organism. Allergy sufferers, for example, are known to have their symptoms exaggerated by electromagnetic fields of a certain frequency.

The balance between health and ill-health, to the extent that it is affected by our electrical environment, depends on the degree of harmony or discord set up in the microstructure vibrations of water. It is therefore to water that we must turn in our search for solutions and remedies for electrical stress symptoms.

---

[1] Tomatis A.A., 1977: *The Conscious Ear*, Centre Tomatis, Paris.

[2] S.C.F Hahnemann, 1810: *Organon der rationellen Heilkunde.*

[3] It is *not* recommended that this be attempted. It is just cited as an example

Chapter 6:
Microstructure information patterns in action

Water's capacity to store and carry information patterns is central to this book.

The foregoing chapters have been mainly concerned with the theoretical background of this comparatively little known aspect of water, and its connection with organisms and the electromagnetic environment of our time. Now, though, we will turn our attention to practical applications which demonstrate the presence and the activity of a water microstructure and its associated information patterns, or 'memory'.

One difficulty encountered in the use of 'structured water', as it is often called, is that electromagnetic fields can, and often do, rapidly destroy such subtle information patterns when water is outside an organism. Water within an organ is to some extent protected by the life-processes themselves, but water in a bottle is very vulnerable to damage. This can result, in practice, in structured water being reduced to nothing more than poor quality tap or distilled water, because it has unwittingly been exposed to strong or persistent electro-magnetic fields at some point in its use. Such water then becomes useless, though people using it (in homeopathic medicine for example) may continue to assume it is having a positive effect.

Despite this caveat, there are a number of processes and applications of water's vibrating information patterns which unequivocally demonstrate that water has a 'memory' quite distinct from the physical substances which it bears, and that it has a vibrating structure of vital importance to the living world. We shall briefly review some of these discoveries and applications, roughly in chronological order.

'Jyomoun-Doki' water storage jars

These pottery jars, whose name derives from the rope pattern in which they were made, were used by Japanese villagers around 2,500 years ago, and unearthed by archaeologists. It is known that villagers stored water in this type of vessel, made of a special clay, because it kept fresh in them for long periods without going stale. We do not now know why the pottery had this property, but the original makers may of course have known what they were doing.

Two Japanese men, Mr Fukazawa and Mr Mori, came across a shard from one of these pots in a museum some years ago, and were very interested in investigating and reviving the process. They both had wide experience in the preparation, cooking and preservation of food, and so they set to work to rediscover the ancient potter's technique. That was 20 years ago. Pottery is much more of a craft than a science, and the possible variations in clay and glaze-mixes, firing times and temperatures, pave the way for endless experimentation.

After much perseverance they came up with a close reproduction of the original pottery. This is a pale, fine-quality stoneware with a dark, matt, chocolate-coloured glaze. This new ceramic has been rechristened with the registered trademark 'BioCeramica'[1] and is now manufactured on a large industrial scale in Japan and sold to a very wide range of industrial, domestic, agricultural, and food processing users. Why? Because it works.

In the presence of this ceramic material, fresh food has a longer shelf-life, fridges keep odour-free, bacterial growth is inhibited, the taste of foods improves, processed food quality improves, recycled water quality improves, powdered substances such as flour do not 'cake'; the list of applications is growing daily. All the reasons behind this ceramic's most useful properties are unclear, but some of the characteristics of the way in which it works have been unravelled.

The pottery has an effect on the water it comes into contact with, or the water in its close proximity. Its presence has the effect of stimulating infra-red generation, that is warmth, in the 'far' infra-red spectrum.[2]

It does not radiate this heat as a hot fire would do, but *stimulates* the generation of energy in the water in its immediate environment. The heat is not radiated from the water either; in other words, it does not get any warmer, but generates an increase in the vibrational activity at a molecular level without causing an increase in temperature.

This change in the vibrational energy of the water gives rise to all the very practical useful effects which are leading people to buy and apply this new material.

One of the characteristics of this ceramic is that it can influence water *without* coming into direct contact with it. An ordinary permanent magnet has a similar property – it can influence a piece of iron that is close but not touching it, through its magnetic field. The field idea has been used many times in the previous pages, and has been defined as a region of space that carries specific properties. This new ceramic has a field around it. This means that a saucer made from BioCeramica has the potential to influence water within its immediate environment, without coming into physical contact. This field has the capacity to stimulate water's molecular vibration in the infra-red region of the spectrum. If there is no water in this field, then the potential remains, but there is no physical change, just as the magnetic field is always round the magnet, but only appears to be active when another magnet or a piece of iron are within its magnetic field.

Because this field round the ceramic affects water, it will affect the water both inside and outside all living organisms that are within its sphere of influence. This, from experience, has various effects on a range of biological functions. The field surrounding this ceramic is therefore a new class of field; it is a field which can influence biological activity.

Physical, manufactured materials that carry such a field are extremely rare, and so such a concept is not common currency. But the practical results are beyond question. The positive effects of this new, or perhaps it should be called 'antique' material, are so apparent and wide-spread that such a field of influence clearly exists, and its presence now supports a rapidly expanding multi-million pound industry.

This example of water's more hidden properties is both ancient and modern; it is old knowledge which has been re-discovered, and applied to solve problems in a completely new situation.

Homeopathy

Samuel Hahnemann published a definitive work in 1810,[3] proposing a quite new approach to medicine, which was generally considered heretical at the time. Almost two centuries later, many in the medical profession still hold the same view about it. Frequently castigated as quackery and nonsense, it has nevertheless persisted and spread world wide. Why? Because it can work. It can work if it is understood, if the practitioner and patient are receptive, and if the general ambience of the environment allows it to work. This environment now involves many factors, including electromagnetic fields, which can block or inhibit the processes of healing embodied in homeopathy.

One of the elements of this practice is the preparation and use of potentised medication, that was described briefly in Chapter 5. The fact that this has been used for two centuries, and now throughout the world, is testimony enough that the preparations can and do have positive effects. One of the obstacles to their general acceptance is the lack of clear understanding of how they work, and the fact that they are not invariably successful. Many experienced practitioners have also reported a decrease in the efficacy of these medications over the last half century.

The preparations consist of water which has been shaken, or 'succussed' in order to transfer the vibrations of a substance to the water. The range of substances available is as wide as the number of mineral and organic substances that can be gathered from any source. Such source materials can be succussed and diluted through a series of steps. The degree of dilution and the number of steps both modify the effects that the final water can have on living organisms – animals as well as people.

Some preparations have quite a low level of dilution and only a few steps, which results in a mixture of dilute physical substance *and* vibrating information patterns in the same preparation. Others will have such high dilution and so many steps that there is no substance left in the water, and it is only 'pure' distilled water with the vibrational imprint of the original substance.

These medications are not very stable, and many of the information patterns naturally degrade in storage. One way in which this can be reduced is to mix the preparation with some alcohol, which is a common practice in a homeopathic pharmacy. Even with this precaution, all information patterns are still very vulnerable to the influence of electromagnetic and magnetic fields. (Electric fields are not such a serious problem, as they may not enter the storage container, depending on frequency.) Exposure of these medications to either of these fields can rapidly degrade the information patterns, which of course renders the medication useless. High levels of these fields can be present in the preparation areas, transport, and storage places, which is one reason for the declining, or at least variable performance of these medicines.

Artificial spring water

Viktor Schauberger was an Austrian forester, and nature lover who gained deep insights into water, particularly in its life in the forest's rivers, aquifers and springs. For generations before him, his family, had lived and cared for the forest, its creatures and its waters. He says of them:

> They relied upon what they saw with their own eyes and
> what they felt intuitively. Above all, they recognised the

inner healing power of water, and understood that water, directed through irrigation channels at night, can yield a significantly greater harvest than the neighbouring meadows and fields. [4]

He lived in the first half of this century and spent much of his time as an apparently maverick hydrological engineer, who decided not to go to University at the age of eighteen, as he observed that it had ruined his elder brother's education. Despite having only nature and his own acute observation as his primary tutors, he managed to achieve extraordinary results with water management that no one has yet been able to successfully reproduce. He learned how to tune machines, flumes, water-courses and pipes to optimise water's latent hydraulic, electric and vibrational properties.

Even in his day – 1930 – natural springs were drying up, and he set to work to generate spring-quality water from tap, river or rain water. He designed an apparatus with an egg-shaped chamber in which water was cooled to 4°C, rotated in a high- speed vortex, and had certain minerals and carbon dioxide added. Many of the design features were critical, such as the special metal alloy of the egg-shaped chamber, and the metal and shape of the rotor, and also the rhythmical change in the speed of rotation. By tuning these and other factors he managed to produce water of exceptional quality, that was reported to taste excellent, cured some ailments and aided recovery from illness.

His machines have not survived, and they have proved impossible to recreate. There are so many factors to tune in order to get these results, and Schauberger seems to have taken the secret with him to the grave. One of the results of the successful design and operation of this equipment is likely to have been an improvement in the microstructure and information patterns of the processed water, which would have given it a renewed spring-like quality.

'Tonsingen' or 'Clay Singing'

Schauberger lived much of his early working life in the Austrian Forest, and knew and respected many local people including farmers. He gave a written report in an essay, *Natural Farming*, of a very unusual meeting with a farmer. This particular farmer was considered more than a little eccentric by his neighbours, but he had the best local harvests. Schauberger went to visit him on one occasion, and found him at his own particular work. He describes this in detail;

> This farmer ploughed in a different way. He also harrowed differently and sowed at times other than those of other farmers. His method of treating crops was also different. In short, he carried out each and every farm process in a unique way. He never went to church; this he would have taken particularly amiss. He was never seen drinking beer with others. Nobody asked him for advice and he never tolerated any arguments from his employees. Those who did not immediately obey him could immediately pack up their goods and chattels and go. Despite this attitude it was seldom that he lost an employee. It was only with his grown son, who attended an agricultural college, and who always thought he knew better, that there was any tension.

> So it happened one day, as darkness was setting in, I came to the farmer's house. I wanted to have a short chat with him. In the courtyard I met the somewhat unsympathetic son and enquired after his father. 'He is at the back of the house – the old one,' he answered with an unfriendly gesture. 'Shout loud enough and he will come.' I went where he pointed, across the threshing floor, and eventually found the old farmer. He was standing in front of a wooden barrel as large as three or four buckets, singing a quaint song. At the same time, he was stirring the contents of the barrel with a large

wooden spoon. It was not really a song he was singing, but rather a musical scale rich in tone, ranging from falsetto to a deep bass. This he did as he bent over the barrel, singing loudly down into it. As he went up the scale, so he rotated the spoon in an anti-clockwise motion. When his voice deepened, so he changed the direction of the rotation of the spoon. I thought to myself that there must be a reason for all this. The farmer did not hear me coming, and after I had watched him for a considerable time, I was curious as to what he was stirring. Unnoticed, I came up to the barrel and glanced inside; there was nothing there except clear water. Eventually the old man noticed me, nodded in reply to my greeting and continued without pause.

My glance alternated between the farmer and the contents of the barrel. With a flick of his hand, he would throw bits of loamy soil into the barrel as he continued to stir the liquid first to the right and then to the left. At the same time he sang quite loudly and not altogether pleasantly into the open container.

'Well,' I thought, 'nothing can last forever'. At last the old man took the giant spoon – it really could be described as a small oar – out of the barrel and muttered, 'So, it's ready for fermenting'.

I nodded, as if to indicate that everything was perfectly clear to me. I nodded again, when the farmer asked me whether I was thirsty and would like a grog of fresh apple juice. So, after the old man had carefully wiped his wet hands on his apron, we went into the house. While he fetched the cool apple juice from the cellar, I walked into the best room. 'Drink up and enjoy it!' With these words he slid the blue-flowered tankard of juice across to me, inviting me to join him.

'Now, do you think as the others do, that I am mad?' asked the farmer. 'You know what you want,' I replied. In the course of our conversation I gradually referred to the series of actions he had just performed and I had noted.

Clay mixed in the cool water with carbonic acid from which the air has been expelled, and then stirred in the right way, will take on a neutral voltage (similar to the effect of well-kneaded loam wrapped in aluminium sheeting).

This neutrally charged water was then sprinkled over newly harrowed and sown fields. The harrow had wooden and not iron teeth. The water eventually evaporated leaving exceedingly fine crystals which carried a negative charge. These crystals attracted rays from all directions and then gave them out again.

Between the geosphere and the atmosphere, a fine membrane, violet in colour, builds up. This skin, acting like a filter, allows rays of the highest value to enter and leave the earth. The down-to-earth farmer called this 'the virgin hymen'. Such a valuble diffusion effect could be obtained, that during the driest part of the year the soil remained cool and moist. By this means, the seed zone between the geosphere and the atmosphere remains at a practically constant temperature of +4°C. At this temperature the crop structure is at its highest potential, while at the same time fructification is relatively passive. As a result of this simple caring for the surface breathing of the earth, an increase in crops of some 30 percent was obtained, compared with where it was not carried out. In the old days this natural breathing action was called 'clay singing'.

Such a labour-intensive and apparently irrational process would be unthinkable in many current agricultural practices, and yet it appeared to produce good results. In the context of the present discussion, it may not seem so strange.

Bach flower remedies

Dr. Edward Bach (1886-1936) was a medical doctor, with a highly respected medical practice off Harley Street, London, in the 1920s. During a dinner party in 1928, he suddenly had a new insight into his dinner companions, as he realised that they fell into several distinct types, and concluded that each type would respond differently to illness. In the same year, he visited Wales and brought back two plants, Mimulus and Impatiens. He prepared these in the way that he was used to preparing vaccines, and prescribed them according to his patients' personality, with immediate success. In the spring of 1930, he closed his practice, and went to Wales to extend his discovery, afterwards settling in Oxfordshire. He spent these years of his life searching for and finding quite new remedies for a number of disorders, particularly emotional and mental disturbance. His method of investigation was very unusual, but very direct. He developed the capacity to induce the symptoms of an illness in himself, and then to search in nature for those flowers which would relieve the symptoms.

Having identified a particular flower species appropriate for particular symptoms, the preparation principle for the remedies was very simple. He took a large bowl of fresh, good quality spring water, and floated a few specimens of the freshly selected flowers on the surface. The bowl was then left in a sheltered place in the midday sunlight for about one hour. Then the flowers were removed and the water mixed with about the same volume of good brandy (alcohol).

He identified 38 different plant species from which to make these preparations. These were used in very small doses, either individually or blended, being diluted in water just before use. These have been in use now for sixty years and have become available in high street chemists. They are still made in the same way, and are mainly used to help stabilise all kinds of emotional and mental problems. One blend which is widely used is marketed under the trade name of 'Rescue Remedy', and many users testify to its immediate help in dealing with the after-effects of shock.

This preparation process transfers the vibrational information patterns from the flower substances to the water, using sunlight as the transfer energy upon the slowly moving myriads of sliding, gently warming water surfaces in the spring water.

Why has it stood the test of time and is still widely used? Because people have found that it works.

Bio-dynamic preparations

The agricultural principles of Bio-Dynamics were set out by Rudolf Steiner in the early 1920s in response to Southern German farmers' concern about the health of their farms. They asked him how to remedy the falling quality of farm produce and the declining health of farm animals, which were evident even at that time, long before current global environmental problems had been recognized as a cause for concern, and before the enormous increase in many environmental pollutants.

One aspect of the new farm management practice that he outlined was to create a set of entirely new preparations for improving the efficacy of manure and compost. These affected the micro-biological decay processes of farmyard manure to improve the health of plants and soil.

One example of these preparations directly demonstrates the action of information patterns in water. Called '501', it is made from finely ground silica. This is placed inside the horn of a cow, and buried in the earth for the summer months. When it is removed in the autumn, the silica powder *appears* to be exactly the same as when it was put into the ground. A very small quantity of this powder is then put into a large container or barrel of fresh, clean spring water and stirred very vigorously first clockwise and then anticlockwise for about one hour. This treated water is then immediately sprayed or sprinkled onto pastures and crops.

This treatment is only one small part of a much more comprehensive land and farm treatment designed to improve the health and vitality of crops and stock. In Australia and New Zealand it has proved extremely effective in countering the effects of drought on large tracts of pasture, where it is sprayed by aircraft. Treated areas show up very clearly against untreated areas. Soil profiles improve as humus and micro-organisms build up in the soil. Stock health improves and vet bills fall. Farmers use it there because it works.

The preparation process seems at first sight to be quite bizarre, but in the light of water microstructure and information patterns, and the importance of form, it begins to make some sense. This preparation process changes the microstructure and the information patterns in the water on the surface of the silica.

But there are, now, serious problems in maintaining the efficacy of this treatment. One of these is the damaging effects of electromagnetic fields during every stage of the process, during stirring if this is done with an electric motor, and particularly immediately after stirring. At this stage, as it is taken for distribution on the land, the water is handled in smaller quantities and is then broken down into single small drops as it is sprayed. In such small amounts, the water structure is particularly vulnerable to rapid breakdown by electromagnetic fields, before it has time to take effect on the plants and micro-organisms. Recent increases in ultra-violet levels in the sunlight and from satellite radiation can also have a rapid and damaging effect on the whole process.

Lightened water

Mr Hachenay, a German, was working on quite standard experiments to research improvement in the quality and structure of concrete. As a part of this development work, he built a piece of apparatus in which water was spun in a very rapid double concentric vortex, inside a specially formed metal chamber. Water that had been through this dynamic process considerably increased the hardness of the concrete made from it. Somehow, the water treatment changed the physical-chemical setting-processes. It is very interesting that a purely physical processing of water can bring about a change in the chemistry of such a hard, durable substance as concrete.

So many discoveries come about through accurate observation of chance phenomena by someone who can see their significance; stainless steel was found quite by accident in a metallurgical laboratory scrap-heap, for example. Something similar happened in this case, when waste water from the vortex apparatus was piped through the lab window onto the flower bed outside. *These plants grew considerably larger than those nearby.*

Investigation into this surprising chance observation, led to a device being manufactured and sold in Germany to improve the quality of water. This change in quality is brought about through the dynamics of the water vortex, which are able to improve the microstructure of the processed water. There is no design provision in this system for imprinting any specific information patterns, so the water may not have any organic benefit, but is a source of improved water structure, which in turn can lead to improved restructuring of information patterns inside a living organism.

Water activation

Johann Grander is an environmentalist, and nature lover who, with others, shares a deep concern for the declining quality of water and the effects that this is having on the living world. He has explored the positive effects that magnetism can have on water, which has led to creating a range of devices that can be connected into a water supply line to improve the quality of the water passing through the system.

In this process, supply water flows over the surface of a specially prepared component containing a fluid with a flow pattern generated by the geometry of the tube through which it flows. The combination of the water movement pattern and the presence of the activated component transfers properties to the water in the supply line.

It is claimed that the inner structure of the water is changed, which has beneficial effects on plants, animals and people. There is also an effect on mineral calcium salts carried in hard water, in that they no longer form a scale in any apparatus that heats water. This treated water even causes a reduction in any scale already present, a property of great benefit to many industrial processing plants.[5]

Water memory in the laboratory

Professor Jacques Benveniste directed a research laboratory in Paris in the 1980s, doing conventional research into a variety of medical problems. He took onto his staff a medical doctor with an additional homeopathic training. They set up a long series of experiments to test the efficacy of homeopathic dilutions. The substance used in the dilution process was an organic substance taken from a goat known as an antiserum. This is known to show a clear reaction with a certain type of human white blood cell, which can easily be detected in an optical microscope.

The antiserum was diluted and shaken in 120 separate stages, resulting in 120 samples of water with decreasing concentrations of the antiserum. According to molecular theory, after about 24 steps there can be no more molecular material of the original substance left in the water. In other words, samples number 25 to 120 contain only distilled water. The effect of these samples on human blood cells was not that expected of distilled water, which ought to have no effect on them. In fact they caused a rhythmical increase and decrease of cell transformation, which can only result from the effects of antiserum on them, even though no physical antiserum was present in the water.

This work was done over a period of seven years, and was duplicated in several other laboratories during this period with the same results. All of these laboratories, particularly the one in Paris, were well established and able to exercise very tight scientific protocol in all their experiments. The publication of this work in the scientific journals in June 1988 caused a furore in the academic scientific world, which rumbled on for years. These experiments unequivocally demonstrate that water has a dynamic memory, even at very high levels of dilution, for which there is no current conventional explanation. These results are a serious challenge to orthodox thinking about the nature of substance and its effects on water; they eventually led to the Paris laboratory being closed down and Jacques Benveniste being castigated because he challenged entrenched views and attitudes, not only in the experiment described, but in a range of similar tests which all confirmed that water has a dynamic memory. [6]

Commercially available systems for structuring water

There are a number of pieces of water treatment equipment available on the open market which are sold for very practical purposes. One proven use is that of re-organising the deposition of calcium carbonate from hard water supplies. Anyone who has lived in a district with hard water knows only too well that deposits of lime scale build up in the kettle. The kettle can be fairly easily cleaned, but the inside of a boiler is a very different matter. The build up of lime deposits in both domestic and commercial boilers is a big and expensive problem.

Several manufacturers offer devices to deal with this that are non-chemical, which appear to bring about a change in the water structure that affects the nature of crystallisation of the calcium carbonate. After treatment, it no longer deposits as hard scale, but forms very fine crystals which do not adhere to the walls of the pipes.

Some of these devices, such as the 'Water King',[7] generate very low-powered impulses to electric coils wrapped round the outside of the main water supply pipe, producing very subtle electric and magnetic fields to bring about a change in the water structure. They may also imprint vibration patterns from the electronic circuit. Other products, such as the 'Care Free' system,[8] use carefully engineered water flow to bring about a change in the water structure. This unit can be fitted to the water main supply pipe so that all the water used flows through the unit. Treated water is reported to eliminate the deposit of limescale, improve plant growth and reduce algal growth in swimming pools.

The 'Leptron Water Treatment Device'[9] comes from Bulgaria, and consists of two very small, low-powered magnets of special construction which, when clamped to the outside of a mains water supply pipe change the structure of the water at an atomic level. The suppliers also claim elimination of calcium scale deposits, softening of the water, and increase in vegetable yields in crops to which treated water has been applied.

Another in-line water mains treatment system comes from Germany, and is called 'Varuna'[10]. This uses a combination of water movement in a particular form, and a specially treated solid silica rod, which imprints the vibrating pattern of the element oxygen into the water. This is claimed to eliminate limescale, improve the quality of food, soften water – therefore reducing the use of detergents and soaps – and to improve plant growth.

The 'Aquator'[11] consists of a small funnel with a permanent magnet structure fitted to the outside, and a small recess into which a sample of material can be inserted. The vibrating pattern from the material is transferred to any water that flows throughout the funnel. It is claimed that all toxic information contained in the water is eliminated, and positive elements are activated. Advertised results include improved plant growth, increased activation of yeast in baking and improved food flavour.

The Ensearch Foundation in Houston, Texas, supply a large range of water that has been pre-treated for use in improving personal health and vitality and treating a number of ailments. Treated water is supplied in sealed tubes, which are placed into water for a short period so that the vibrations from the sealed tube are transferred to the body of water into which it has been placed. A very interesting aspect of these devices is that the water in the tube has only been 'treated' by the consciousness of a single human being, Ann Johnson. The reported results from users are impressive. (If this sounds a little unlikely, there are clear reports of water that is treated in this way showing a change in the infra-red transmission spectrum.)

Another man who has made use of the vibration properties of water is Roland Plocher in southern Germany. He has imprinted the vibration pattern of oxygen onto silica powder and used this very successfully to improve the rate and quality of the bacterial breakdown of cow and pig manure in liquid form, which is a great problem for intensive cattle and pig farmers. The addition of some of this material to a large quantity of liquid manure reduces the time taken for the normal breakdown of the material to a useable manure. Many farmers report good results. It is interesting to note, though, that in regions where the electromagnetic environment is highly active, this process does not work satisfactorily. It seems that both mains power and radio frequency fields inhibit the process. It also does not work on a small laboratory scale, but only in quantities above about 500 litres.

These examples all indicate that water can accept structure and information patterns which can affect a number of mineral and organic processes. It is important to distinguish between these two. Structuring the water has to do with *changing* the microstructure of the water. Information patterns, on the other hand, are vibrating patterns *within* the microstructure. Some of the above examples create a changed water structure, others imprint vibration patterns, and still others may do both at the same time. Microstructure and the vibration patterns that they hold are two quite distinct aspects of water's properties.

Water with a poor microstructure can only hold a limited range of information patterns, whereas a water with a complex microstructure has the potential to hold a far wider range of vibrations. In the above commercial examples, it is not clear which aspect of the process is being applied in each case, and it cannot be assumed that the resulting treated water is automatically beneficial for all applications. What is beneficial for chemical processes may not necessarily be suitable for human consumption.

In the examples given in this chapter, one of water's more subtle and less obvious properties has been put to use by a range of people – from the experienced, intuitive farmer to the professional rational scientist. Across this spectrum of experience, the findings are the same, bearing clear evidence of an important property of water in relation to the organic world and the way in which it works. Recognition of this fact throws some light on the effects of electric, electromagnetic and magnetic fields on water and organisms in the new vibrating environment in which we and nature are now embedded.

One more example of a somewhat different kind shows the connection between the vibration patterns of water and influences from far beyond the boundaries of the immediate earth environment. This is the work of Professor Piccardi and C. Capel-Boute.[12] Piccardi worked in Italy from the 1930s to the 1960s and Capel-Boute on into the 1990s. Piccardi was a chemist, and his painstaking work in examining the rates at which certain chemical reactions proceed, challenged the prevailing view that all chemical reactions are independent of their surroundings, and that water is just the carrier of the reaction but does not in any way control it. This led to the conclusion that reproducibility of results in certain chemical and some biological reactions is a myth. You cannot do the same experiment day after day and get the same results.

He arranged for trials to be duplicated in 30 different locations from the arctic to the antarctic over a period of many years and got confirmation of his results from all the other researchers. The trials involved hundreds of thousands of tests. The results are very significant, and there are two key elements:

- Chemical reactions were influenced by the pre-treatment of water used. (Pre-treatment with a mercury-filled glass tube which was used to stir the water before performing the experiment.)

- The rate of the chemical reaction showed considerable variation, which demonstrated a correlation with the changing, relative position of the sun and the earth.

He attributed this variation to the reaction of the treated water to subtle variations in the electric, electromagnetic and magnetic fields of the earth and their modulation by the sun. Changes in the water's structure altered this relationship.

This is very significant, for it means that even at the test-tube level, the microstructure of water is open to the natural electromagnetic environment and **its variations,** and can influence the rate of the chemical reaction. It is interesting to note that much of this work was done around the 1950s when the electromagnetic environment was far less disturbed than it is now, and that similar experiments are now far more difficult to reproduce.

At every turn, man-made electromagnetism demonstrates its fundamental conflict with the forces and rhythms of organic life. But as we have seen in this chapter, there are ways in which life-forces can be strengthened to counteract this influence. Let us now look once more at water's potentially life-enhancing properties.

---

[1] BioCeramica is a registered trademark of LOE Group of Companies or BioCeramica Ltd.

[2] A wavelength of 5 to 50 microns.

[3] S.C.F Hahnemann, 1810, *Organon der rationellen Heilkunde*.

[4] Olaf Alexanderson 1990, *Living Water,* Gateway Books

[5] These products are marketed by Ecolife Technology Enterprises, BC Canada.

[6] Davenas E. Benveniste, J. et al. 1988, 'Human Basophil Degranulation Triggered by Very Dilute Antiserum Against IgE', in *Nature,* vol. 333, June 1988, p816.

Also: Benveniste J. 1994, *Heretic,* a BBC2 documentary shown on 6/2/94

[7] 'Water King' is supplied by Lifescience Products Ltd, UK

[8] 'Carefree' products supplied by Care-Free Water Products, California, USA.

[9] 'Leptron' devices supplied by The Grain of Wheat, Surrey, UK.

[10] 'Varuna' supplied by Lightconnect, Berlin, Germany.

[11] 'Aquator' is supplied by Harmonology, Glasgow, UK.

[12] Piccardi G., 1959, *On the Structure of Water and the Influx of Low-frequency Electromagnetic Fields,* La Ricreca Scientifica 29:1252.

Also: Piccardi G., 1962, *The Chemical Basis of Medical Climatology,* Springfield.

Also: Piccardi G., Capel-Boute C., 1972, *The 22-year solar cycle and chemical tests,* in Journal Interdiscip. Cycle Res. 3:413-417.

Chapter 7:
Life-Rhythms and Water

Besides physical and electromagnetic vibrations, there is a third and quite distinct group of patterns of change that find expression in the organic world. These are the *rhythms* which show themselves in the multitude of organic processes in any organism. They are not identical with the physical processes themselves, but are dynamic time patterns which orchestrate and govern the physical processes, such as heartbeat or breathing.

Opinion is sharply divided, polarised even, as to whether organic rhythms have their origin *within* the material substances of the living organism itself, or whether they form a *separate and independent* set of dynamics – known as the life-forces – which organize and regulate it.

This is the nub of the issue surrounding the two methodologies of investigation mentioned in the introduction to this book: instrumental data versus direct individual experience. Whether the regulating forces of the organic world are part of, and of the same nature as, the physical substances of which it is built; or whether they are of an independent, though intimately related, nature. This is a question of primary importance. If the latter is the case, then a whole new area of investigation – of studying and understanding health, disease, and ecological balance – can open up.

Our work and experience quite clearly supports the second view.

Several decades of research into the origin of these regulating time patterns within the substances and complexities of the DNA molecule, and elsewhere in the organic substances, have failed to find any satisfactory origin. What is clear from such investigations, though, is that there are very precise and complex biochemical processes at work within the tissues, including many electrical activities – particularly at cell boundaries and tissue surfaces – which are vital for the implementation of these rhythmic processes.

Electrical and magnetic forces and their variable time-patterns are accepted as non-physical forces, because they can so clearly have controlling effects on physical substances. When the electrical supply is turned off, the radio, hoover or computer stops working, and they are then commonly referred to as 'dead'. All the components of the machine may be in order, but without the activating electrical energy nothing happens.

Likewise, when the life-rhythms stop in an organism, it is considered to be dead. All the tissues may be in perfect condition at the moment of death, and yet the fact that rhythmic activity has ceased and does not start again of its own accord means, of course, that life is no longer present. The unexplained occurrence of cot-death is a tragic example of this.

The rhythmic processes of life in any organism are very intimately integrated into the tissues, but such close, interwoven co-operation does *not* necessarily mean that they are of the same nature, and simply generated by the substances of the tissues themselves.

In music, the time structure is the creation of the composer, and is re-created by the musicians each time the piece is played. This temporal 'architecture' exists quite independently of the individual pitch of the notes which form the melody. In order for the music to come to expression, all elements must be present and integrated into a whole. In living processes the same seems to be true. The right substance must be present in the right place, at the right time, in the right concentration for any specific process to take place. In order for this to happen, it must be organised; and the organisation requires a constant source of information and a dynamic set of forces to activate it.

There are, then, three quite distinct but interwoven types of time-varying patterns that affect living organisms. They have their origins in:

- Vibrations from the electrical, electromagnetic and magnetic fields.
- Vibrations from physical substances.
- Rhythmic expression of life-forces (life-rhythms).

Water as a physical substance is affected and influenced by all three groups of forces and time patterns **(diagram 16)**. This in turn means that any living organism is subject to the influences of all three types of force. How does this happen? We will look at each of the three types in turn.

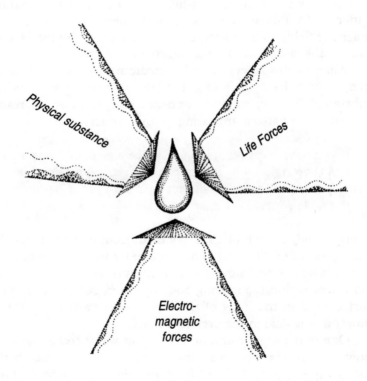

Diagram 16: Three forces acting on water

Earlier, we outlined the microstructure of water, and its ability to receive and act as a store for vibrational information. This is built from individual molecules of water, which have an electrical polarisation – one side is positive and the other negative. The detailed architecture of the various different microstructure types is not yet known clearly, so the differences in the electrical properties are not clear. What is certain, though, is that the microstructure forms retain some quite specific electrical properties. These electrical positive and negative charges mean that any external electrical or magnetic field can generate electrical forces on the structure, because it carries its own electric field. These forces, in turn, can affect the vibrational state of the form, which is the carrier of information patterns. In this way, the electrical, magnetic and electro-magnetic fields all have access to the microstructure forms, and can modify stored vibrational information patterns.

Water is also a very sensitive medium to *mechanical* vibrations, which have their origin in the movement of physical substances. The slightest tremor near a body of water will result in a vibration pattern appearing on the surface.

If you have a strong pulse, and place a glass of water on a not too rigid table, it is possible to see the pulse in the vibrations of the water surface by putting your hand on the table somewhere near the glass.

Every sound, every footfall, every earth tremor, every breath of wind sets water vibrating. These are external forces acting on water. When water moves, it also frequently sets up its *own* vibrations within the moving body of water, both on the water surface and in the body of the liquid. One particular type of movement is vital in the present context.

One of the most common forms that water creates when it moves is the **vortex.** This dynamic shape has intrigued bath-tub dwellers young and old for generations, and occurs quite naturally in many, many situations. Watch any slowish river: languid vortices appear, pirouette across the surface and quietly melt into the background movement, in an endless procession. In turbulent rapids, myriads of minute tumbling vortices are generated in the chaotic, cascading water. Stir a cup of tea, and watch the surface vortex speed up and slow down in rhythmic succession as the vortex slows. The vortex is so common that it can almost be thought of as one of water's 'signatures'.

The anatomy of the vortex structure shows several key features. The real dynamics of this form begin to become apparent when one views the vortex from the side, through a transparent tank. The surface between the air and the spinning water generates three clearly defined sections (**diagram 17**). The top section, 'A', is very smooth, and appears stretched like a drum. The centre section, 'B', has a surface that is twisted, like a piece of coarse rope. The very tip of the form, 'C', appears smooth to the naked eye, but is extremely unstable. The whole form rotates very slowly at the top outer surface, but with accelerating speed as the water approaches the centre at point 'C', where the rotational speed becomes very high.

The body of water immediately below the surface of sections 'A' and 'B' is also spinning but not quite as fast as the surface immediately above it. Water always moves in sliding surfaces, rather like a pack of cards being fanned out, where each card slides over both its adjacent neighbours. There is not really just one surface where the water meets the air in a vortex, but innumerable, nested, closely packed, vortex-shaped surfaces all sliding over each other with decreasing rotational speed from the surface. Each surface has a highly organised dynamic form, similar but not identical to the water-air surface.

Section 'B' is a very dynamic form. The twisted surface is never stable, but is constantly expanding and contracting, and carrying a large variety of vibrations on its surface. As well as the clearly visible rope-like twist, which rapidly oscillates up and down, there are many fine waveforms on the surface of the twist. These appear to be be formed and move at random, but within the apparently chaotic variation of frequencies there are patterns of order. For example, there are periods where one particular type of vibration dominates, which then gives way to

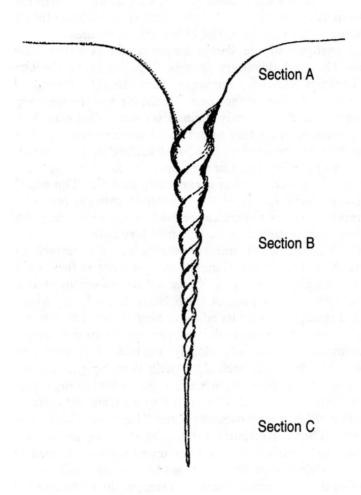

Diagram 17: Water vortex

another; and such alternations and transitions can have a daily rhythm, for example. This section of the vortex form is a very sensitive surface for vibrations – not those mechanically generated from external physical surroundings, but those which arise within the dynamics of the water itself and the form of its surfaces. The surface of water shows vibrations as ripples, but these patterns spread into the body of the liquid, and affect the other sliding water surfaces – though with decreasing intensity from the surface.

So in the basic properties of the water vortex structure, three vital elements can be identified:

- The overall form or shape of the vortex
- The sliding surfaces in the water
- The vibrations

The fact that this common water form combines these three elements is of critical importance for its relation to all three types of forces mentioned above, for it is through this form that the water microstructure can receive new information patterns. This is how the process of succussion used in the preparation of homeopathic medications works. The process of shaking generates turbulence which consists of myriads of tiny vortices. These vortices in water in which a substance is dissolved, imprint the subtance's vibrational pattern into the water.

The third of these forces or time-patterns – the *life rhythms* – have access to water through a combination of two distinct components. One is the water information patterns in the microstructure, and the other is the form of the surfaces which surround them.

One of the most elementary and striking phenomena of the living world is that all organisms are constructed from surfaces which have water in and around them. Whether it is at the micro-level of individual cell structure, or complete organisms such as an orange, they all consist of abundant organic tissues in which one set of surfaces nestle inside another, which is in turn inside another... and so on, like a Russian Babushka doll. Comparatively few organic tissues are truly three-dimensional in the sense of a solid, the vast majority consisting of a very thin sheet or membrane of material formed into a three-dimensional surface, such as a cell wall, or an animal's skin.

The material surrounding the surfaces – water – bears a host of dissolved materials *and* a complex microstructure with its associated information patterns. Even water, which is a three-dimensional substance, generates myriads of surfaces as soon as it moves, and the majority of water in an organism is in some form of movement, even if it is slow.

It is the tissue and water surfaces, dissolved physical substances, and water microstructures which are the vital elements connecting the organic world to the rhythmic life processes.

Any organism is in communication with these life forces through a combination of its many surface forms and the information patterns held in the water of its tissues. If the form is healthy and is therefore the 'right' shape, then it can act as a form of resonator. If it is not correctly tuned, then it cannot resonate. The important question of form and its relation to vibrations – in other words, the whole question of whether life-forces are able to penetrate the organism in a health-giving way – will be dealt with in much more detail in the next chapter.

Chapter 8:
The Energy Vortex

Form is one of the primary characteristics of the world around us. Many things have a clear outer boundary or surface. Bricks, leaves and pencils have very sharp clear boundaries. Clouds, flames and smells have less distinct edges. Although the forms of the organic world are often very characteristic of a particular species or function, the purpose of many is, nevertheless, not immediately apparent. Flowers are a typical example. They are very beautiful, but *why* are they the shape that they are? Do natural shapes have a purpose? In our researches into the nature of form and its relation to vibrations in water we have uncovered a property of certain forms that is of critical importance.

Certain types of form have the capacity to generate a vortex of energy around themselves.

This is quite a complex phenomenon, and breaks new ground in the understanding of form. The critical element is a particular characteristic of certain types of form very common in the organic world.

This key characteristic can only be exactly stated by using a particular type of mathematics, called projective geometry. For those who would like to understand the mathematics of this in detail, it is very well presented in a book by Lawrence Edwards titled *The Vortex of Life*.[1]

This property of surfaces in question concerns transformation; and an important aspect of understanding anything undergoing transformation is to ask ourselves what remains *unchanged*. To take a trivial example: on holiday you might see someone coming towards you wearing beach shorts, sunglasses and flip-flops, and in these unfamiliar surroundings you fail to recognize him. As he walks past, you think to yourself, 'I'd know that voice anywhere'. Sure enough, though everything else has changed, you can identify his voice as belonging to a different, familiar context. The voice is the one feature that did not change in an otherwise totally different situation.

To take a more mathematical example: if you multiply any number you like to think of by two, a very simple arithmetic transformation results. What number can you think of that remains unchanged when you multiply it by two? Answer: zero. Twice nought is nought. This singles out nought as a very different sort of number from all the other numbers that you can think of. Mathematicians are always very interested in elements that remain *unchanged* in any transformation procedure.

The critical property of the forms we are considering is that their surfaces remain unchanged when a particular geometric transformation is performed on them. When this transformation is applied to most forms they will change their shape, perhaps even dramatically. This is a mathematical process, but, interestingly, it appears to have a direct practical relation to the world of forms around us. These surfaces that remain unchanged are called 'pathcurve surfaces', a term coined by their mathematical discoverers Felix Klein and Sophus Lie late last century.

The requirements for a form to have a pathcurve surface are quite demanding. If you were carefully to model an egg-shape in plasticine, the chances of it being a pathcurve form would be very slight. A chicken, on the other hand, *always* lays eggs that are pathcurves. Eggs come in many shapes and sizes but they nearly always meet this special form criterion. Eggs, shells, bones, buds and many other organic forms all fall into this category of pathcurve forms, and have been found to very accurately embody this special contour characteristic. Man-made forms, on the other hand, are only pathcurves if they are specially designed to be so. This type of form very rarely arises by accident, and yet appears to be one of the 'design criteria' of organic forms.

It is these pathcurve forms that generate an energy vortex. If the form is even slightly distorted then the vortices do not appear. Since this type of form does not often arise by accident, this means that such vortices generally only occur around living forms. This kind of vortex is drawn in **diagram 18**. (see Appendix 2 for full diagram).It is not just a single surface, but consists of a number of concentric shells. The axis of this vortex set is quite independent of the orientation of the physical form. In other words, rotating the form does not rotate the axis of the vortices – the vertical axis always remains vertical. Although these forms and therefore their vortices abound in nature, we are not normally aware of them as they are not apparent to our everyday senses. The same can be said, of course, for magnetism.

This brings us to a rubicon, and it is the one about methodology referred to in the introduction. *Electricity and life are different. The forces of electricity and magnetism do not fall into the same class of forces as the life forces which maintain all the complex rhythms of a living organism.* In order to explore and understand the electrical world it is essential to use some form of detection instrument. This has given rise to a wide range of measuring instruments that are vital for sensing what is happening in the relation between the electromagnetic forces and the physical world – without them we would have no idea of what is going on there. Yet this has been so successful that people are now very disinclined to accept or contemplate anything that has *not* been measured or quantified in some way, by means of one kind of instrument or another.

The boundary between the electrical forces and the physical world is not the same boundary as the one existing between the life forces and the physical world.

Because these are two different boundaries with quite different characteristics, the process of exploration of the two must necessarily also be different.

The technique for exploring any boundary between differing forces is to find something which will be sensitive to both sets of forces that meet at the boundary. In the case of electricity and magnetism this is an electromechanical device

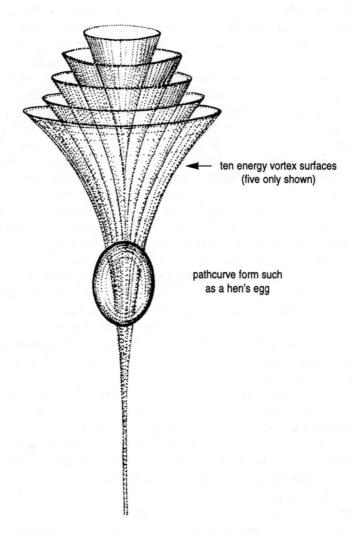

Diagram 18: Energy vortex over a pathcurve form

that incorporates both the forces of electromagnetism and those of physical mechanics. This is the basis of all such instrumentation.

When we come to the boundary between the physical forces and the life forces, these instruments are useless. A new instrument is needed; one that incorporates both the life forces and the forces of the physical mechanical world. This means that only living organisms can be used, for only they combine these two sets of forces. This has given rise to the use of 'biosensors'. So the breathing rate of a fish or the light emission of a bacterium are used to indicate how the life processes react to a toxin in water, for example. It is only possible to sense like with like, so living organisms can be used to indicate changes in the relation of the life forces to the physical world.

The vortices over pathcurve forms cannot, therefore, be sensed with normal instruments, but only with a biosensor, for they exist at the boundary between the physical and the life forces. *The biosensor in this case is the human being,* making use particularly of the life forces that are active in the hands. This vortex form can be sensed with the bare hands if they are sensitive enough, and if you know what you are looking for – such sensitivity is of a very similar kind to that developed by dowsers and healers. The boundaries and dynamics of this vortex can be objectively felt as surely as one feels the surface of a liquid. This is a subtle process, but one that with care and training can become quite objective and reliable; as reliable at this boundary as the electric meter is at the electrical boundary. Such an objective sensing is not a common capacity, being quite difficult to develop. Continuous practice with subtle movements of the hand – particularly the right hand – near pathcurve forms, can result in a new, refined, non-physical sense of touch. The experience is similar to touching a veil made of some very thin and fine material.

We have done a great deal of investigation into the behaviour and properties of this vortex, and the results open an area of new understanding for the way in which the vibrations in water work, and how they are affected by electricity.

In our researches it seemed at first sight as though just the *form* of any material, if it was a pathcurve, would generate a vortex. We have made such forms in a variety of materials such as concrete, silicone rubber and acrylic resin, and all have shown this vortex property. On much closer examination, though, it was found that the material of the surface itself was not critical, but the water carried by that surface. All materials at room temperature carry a very thin film of water on them. Even things that look perfectly dry bear this water on their surfaces, and it is this which is the active element.

So the key criterion for a vortex to be generated is that water should be formed with a pathcurve surface. It is water that is vital to this vortex process.

This vortex is not static as drawn in the diagram. It undergoes a wide variety of change in form and strength, involving a number of cycles. Some changes take place in very rapid cycles over a period of a few seconds. Others take minutes or hours. Some longer cycles take a fortnight, a month or a year. The two-week and four-week rhythm has been found to be directly connected to the phases of the moon, particularly new and full moon, but the effects of these vary depending on the time of year. So a very complicated picture of a dynamic process surrounding pathcurve forms – that is, living forms – begins to emerge.

To complicate things still further, it appears that different forms generate different vortex dynamics. The outer form of the energy vortex in two different physical forms, such as an egg and a flower bud, may both appear to be the same, but the inner dynamics are different. This throws a very interesting light on the function of forms in nature. Different forms generate subtly different vortices. This is important because these vortices are connected with the microstructure and vibration patterns in water, and these vary greatly.

In Chapter 9 we will look at devices we have designed to provide protection against electromagnetic disturbances. One of these, used on trees, consists of small pathcurve egg forms cast with silica, which carries a particular microstructure and vibrating information pattern. Such a device brings together two interacting elements: the vortex structure and the vibrations carried by the water on the silica, (for silica is always covered by a film of water). The vortex above the form flows downwards vertically and passes through the egg from top to bottom. As it passes through the egg it also passes through the water on the silica. The vibration pattern on the silica is transferred to the dynamic of the vortex and is carried down below the form of the egg, as shown in **diagram 19**. This means that the information pattern can be transmitted vertically downwards, carried by the vortex stem.

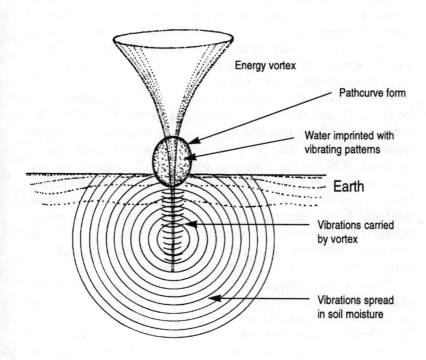

*Diagram 19: Transfer of vibrations from water
into the soil by an energy vortex*

When the stem of the vortex meets another water surface, the information pattern is propagated into the water. This means that if such an egg is simply placed onto damp soil, the water in the soil propagates the information pattern in all directions. This effectively sets up a field of vibrations identical to those held on the silica in the egg. The distance over which it is transmitted depends on a number of conditions, but typically extends up to a few yards. The practical application and results of this process will be discussed in the following chapter.

The vortex above a form has a direction of flow vertically downwards, but it also has a direction of clockwise rotation (looking down onto the vortex from above). All pathcurve forms, under normal conditions, appear to give the same direction of rotation. It is as well to remember that the vortex is generated by the water on the form and not by the form itself, so the water on the surface of the form normally gives a clockwise direction to the vortex.

There is one condition where the direction of rotation can be reversed, and that is in a vibrating magnetic field. If a pathcurve egg form is brought into a mains frequency magnetic field, for example, then the direction of rotation will tend to be reversed. Whether or not it is reversed will depend on the strength of the magnetic field. Since its natural rotational direction is clockwise, this is a very significant change. A magnetic field also brings about a second important change. The vortex tends to contract to a very narrow stem both above and below the form **(diagram 20)**. This gives rise to an anticlockwise rotating column passing through the form.

Both of these changes are brought about by the water on the surface of the form, which is now set vibrating by the frequency of the magnetic field. It appears that this is a very significant factor in electromagnetic stress. In any living organism there will be a multitude of pathcurve surfaces, all of which naturally have clockwise vortices over them. If the organism is affected by a vibrating magnetic field, the vortices will narrow as the strength of the field increases, until a point is reached where the rotation reverses and the vortex is reduced to a very narrow column.

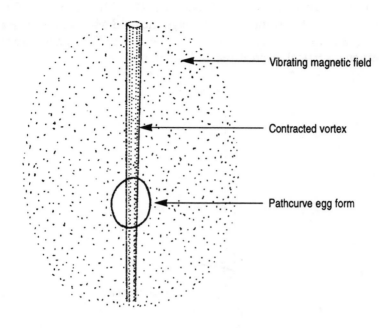

Vibrating magnetic field

Contracted vortex

Pathcurve egg form

*Diagram 20: Contracted energy vortex
in a vibrating magnetic field*

There is another situation in which a very narrow anticlockwise vortex stem is generated, and that is over electromagnetic coils. Most electrical apparatus is hidden in boxes or cabinets so that few people have any idea what is inside. One of the common components of electromagnetic equipment is a coil of copper wire which, when connected to the mains supply, generates a vibrating magnetic field. This magnetism is what drives all electric motors for example – even the Intercity trains are pulled along by such magnets in the engine. Every telephone, fax machine, photocopier, vacuum cleaner, washing machine, TV, computer, fluorescent light, lamppost and transformer all have their coils of wire hidden away out of sight. Every single coil brings about a degenerate, vertical, column-like, anticlockwise rotating vortex **(diagram 21)**. The strength of it depends on the strength of the magnetic field within the coil. As with the vortex over the egg, the axis of the column always remains vertical, even if the coil is rotated.

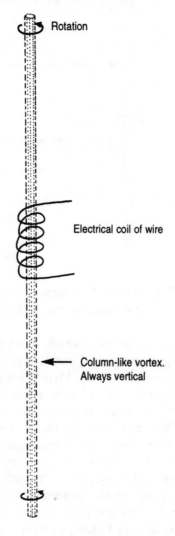

Diagram 21: Column vortex over an electric coil of wire

The magnetic fields generated by the coils in machinery diminish very rapidly as you move away from the equipment, so it is usually assumed that the effect of any magnetic field is confined to the region close to the machine. This is quite true for the *direct* effect of the magnetic field itself, but not for the column vortex it generates, which reaches vertically far above and below the coil and penetrates almost everything, carrying vibrations from the electric supply.

This gives quite a new perspective on the disturbances caused by electrical apparatus, as the *effect* of the magnetic field can now be seen to reach beyond the field itself **(diagram 22)**.

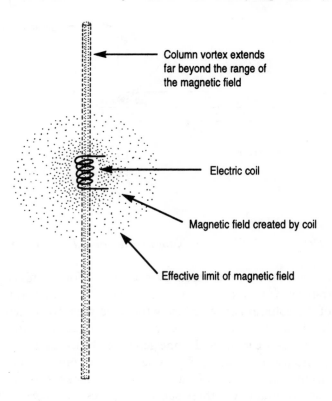

Column vortex extends far beyond the range of the magnetic field

Electric coil

Magnetic field created by coil

Effective limit of magnetic field

Diagram 22: Column vortex of disturbance extending beyond the magnetic field of an electric coil of wire

In practice this means that a fluorescent light, for example, which contains quite a large coil of wire making quite an intense local magnetic field, has in addition a vertical column of vibrations which reaches far above and below the fitting **(diagram 23)**. This column penetrates floors, ceilings and everything in its way. The *magnetic field* created by the coil of wire would have an extremely low value at floor level under the fitting, whereas the *column of disturbance* is quite strong. This disturbance cannot be registered on conventional magnetic field meters, but it nevertheless has an effect on organic forms and all pathcurve surfaces.

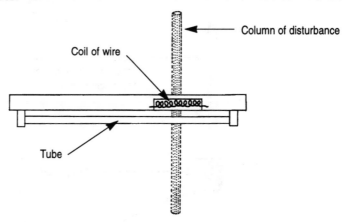

Diagram 23: Coil and column vortex in a fluorescent light fitting

As with the previous vortex over pathcurve forms, this column can transfer its vibrations to a water surface if the water is in the path of the column above or below the apparatus that is generating it. If this water is in the tissues of a living organism, two conflicting processes are generated – one generated by the pathcurve surfaces in the tissues rotating clockwise, and a second coming from the electromagnetic coil of wire rotating anticlockwise – which creates a stress situation in these subtle dynamics. This means that if you are sitting directly under the magnetic coil of a fluorescent light, a stress situation is set up in your body.

To take another specific example: a power transformer is a very powerful magnetic machine, which generates strong magnetic fields within the apparatus. Such transformers are a very common and essential part of our electrical distribution system. Although they generate a very strong magnetic field, this decreases very rapidly as you move away from the case of the machine. At a distance of only a few yards there would be little to register on a magnetic field meter. In addition to the magnetic field, a trans-former creates a very strong column of disturbance above and below the transformer, which reaches down into the ground. This is not magnetic. If the column meets some water that is moving, then the disturbance is propagated along the line of flow of the water, both with and against the flow **(diagram 24)**.

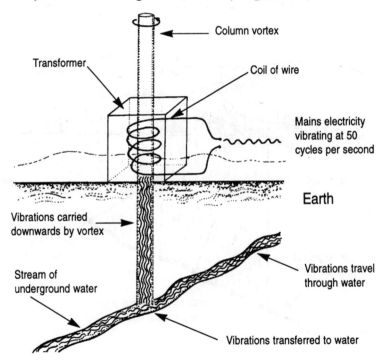

Diagram 24: Transfer of vibrations by a
transformer to water in the ground

Water always makes surfaces when it moves, and it is these surfaces that are able to receive and propagate the disturbance. The result of this is, in effect, that the column of disturbance is spread out along the line of flow of the ground water, and appears as a continuous plane above the water, even at ground level **(diagram 25)**. This disturbance can travel a considerable distance from the transformer, far far beyond the range of the transformer's magnetic field.

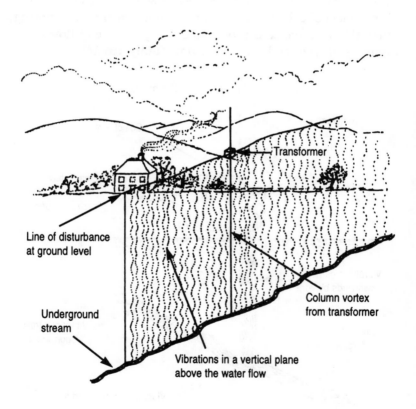

Diagram 25: A transformer creating a line of disturbance from ground water

If this line of water-flow crosses a second stream of water in or on the surface of the ground, the disturbance is also transferred to the second stream and propagated along its line of flow. A network of lines can thus be created at the surface by a single powerful source, such as a transformer or heavy electric motor. In certain geological strata, water flowing in the ground is a very common occurrence, and so the phenomenon described above is also quite common in many areas **(diagram 26)**.

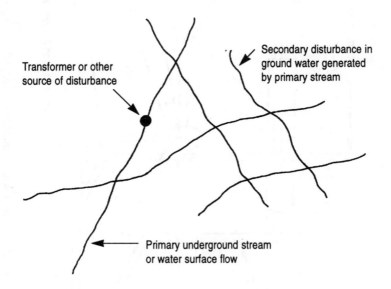

Transformer or other source of disturbance

Secondary disturbance in ground water generated by primary stream

Primary underground stream or water surface flow

Diagram 26: Ground plan of a network of lines of disturbance on the surface, generated from one source such as a transformer

Such lines are often thought to be natural ley lines, earth energy lines or lines of geopathic stress, when in fact they are the direct result of some heavy industrial electromagnetic equipment. The result – as picked up by a dowser – will be very similar at the ground surface, but the origins of the two phenomena are quite different. It is a fact that our use of powerful electromagnetic machines has generated a very extensive network of disturbance that usually goes unnoticed, but which can nevertheless have a

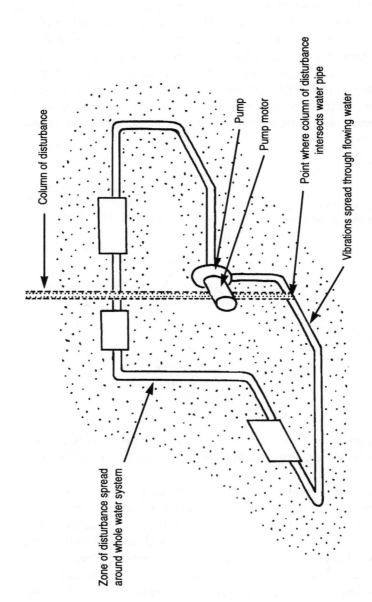

Diagram 27: Disturbance in a house caused by a central heating system

Column of disturbance

Pump

Pump motor

Point where column of disturbance intersects water pipe

Vibrations spread through flowing water

Zone of disturbance spread around whole water system

detrimental effect on health. The strength (or even any appearance at all) of these lines, is directly dependent on the electrical load on the originating equipment, and this often follows daily and annual patterns as electrical demand varies. In practice this means that the disturbance can come and go, as can the effects that it causes. More specific details about this can be found in Appendix 1.

Another very common situation in which an electromagnetic motor can cause a disturbance is in a central heating system. Most heating systems use water which is circulated through a network of radiators by an electric pump. The pump itself is driven by an electric motor which contains a number of coils of wire, which in turn make strong electromagnets. Above and below each of these magnetic coils a column of disturbance is generated when the pump is running. If this column happens to intersect one of the pipes or any other moving water in the system, then the disturbance is transferred to the water and propagated round the whole water network. This sets up a series of zones of disturbance in the building above and below the pipes and at other places, due to a complex process of interference. As with the other examples above, this effect reaches far beyond the range of the magnetic field of the motor which is only very local round the machine. We have found this to be quite a common source of serious disturbance in houses and commercial buildings **(diagram 27)**.

A central heating system can also be affected by a line of disturbance coming from the ground, as described above. If the disturbance crosses a central heating pipe in which water is flowing, then, as with ground water, the disturbance will be transferred to the whole water system in the pipes.

All of these various zones of disturbance are generated by the effects of coils of wire which are used to create electromagnets. In every case the primary cause is the same: namely that a column-like, degenerate, anti-clockwise vortex forms, which appears to be an important component of electromagnetic stress.

Electronic equipment creates a very different effect from the above. There are a wide variety of electronic machines in intermittent or constant use in almost every type of building. By far the most common and complicated in terms of the fields generated are the TV and the computer – the exposure time of many people, particularly children, to these two machines, is now second only to the time that they spend asleep, so it would be prudent to be as alert as possible about the effect they have. This issue has many levels, but we are only concerned here with the field effects generated, and how to do something about them.

All TVs and the majority of personal computers use a cathode ray tube to display the images. This is a highly sophisticated glass bottle lying on its side, containing a few carefully engineered pieces of metal and a high vacuum. The TV screen that carries the display is the bottom of the bottle, seen end-on, which is coated on the inside with a material that produces light when it is bombarded with cathode rays. These rays can only exist in a vacuum, where they are made to move in a series of horizontal lines over the screen, generating patterns of light which we see as pictures. In order to do this, strong electric and magnetic fields are generated inside and around the tube, together with very specific waveforms in the electric circuits. The vacuum tube has carefully shaped magnetic coils around it to create the required form of magnetic field.

In order to supply the high voltages needed for the tube, a mains supply transformer is built into the TV set or computer. This again contains a number of coils of wire and generates a magnetic field in just the same way as any other coil. In a TV these, in conjunction with the tube, are the main sources of disturbance.

In most computers, in addition to these components, there is a hard disk for storage of information. The hard disk consists of a flat rigid disk a few inches in diameter which is coated with a thin layer of magnetic material. This magnetic surface is imprinted with magnetic patterns which correspond to the data that have to be stored, and is driven round by a small electric motor all the time the computer is switched on. For many computers now, this means twenty-four hours a day, as suppliers recommend for technical reasons that they are never turned off.

The computer and the TV introduce two elements into the electrical processes which are very different from those so far discussed. These are the cathode ray and the waveform of electricity. While all mains supplies and radio transmissions use a sinewave pattern for electrical processes – so that most of the disturbances approximately follow this pattern – the generation of cathode rays, and their management in the tube and the electronic circuits of computers, produces quite different patterns of electrical activity **(diagram 28)**. These patterns are transferred to the fields emanating from the TV and the computer.

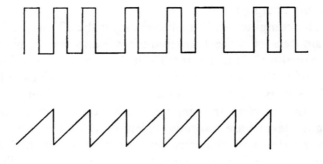

Diagram 28: Television waveforms

The various electrical and magnetic activities generate a very complex field structure round both the TV and the computer, and all three of the fields so far discussed – the electric, magnetic and electromagnetic – are present. This means that the three fields are present simultaneously in the same space, each with its own shape and structure. The anatomy of these fields will vary from one installation to another, but the basic pattern is the same. Colour TV and computer monitors use far higher voltages in the cathode ray tube than monochrome displays, which means that their fields have a higher intensity and extend further from the set.

The *electric* field is mainly generated by the activity at the screen, which can have a high static voltage after a set has been in use for a while. This can be felt on a colour TV by touching the screen, which can give a crackling sound and a slight electric shock. There is no risk from these shocks themselves, but the field from this electric charge spreads out, in front and to the side of the screen, though with a rapidly reducing intensity as you move away from the set. This field is easily screened using an add-on screen and glare protector, which eliminates it.

Magnetic fields generated by the coils are not strong, but spread out around the machine in an asymmetric pattern depending on the layout of the transformers, disk and motor. Again these decrease rapidly in intensity as you move away from the equipment.

The computer and to a lesser extent the TV are both radio transmitters of quite high frequency radio waves, which are *electromagnetic* in nature. TV license dodgers are found by listening to the radio frequency transmissions from each TV set. High security computer operators have the problem of making the activities of their computers safe from bugging, as some bugging devices are just radio receivers which can listen to and interpret the radio transmissions automatically made by every computer. Computers actually transmit all their electrical activity out into the space around them, generating an electromagnetic field. This is of very low intensity, but is continuous, and contains certain frequencies and frequency patterns. This travels a very long way in all directions, but also reduces in intensity as you move away from the machine.

In addition to these three fields, the various components of the TV and computer monitor form regions in which there is a disturbance generated by degenerate vortices as described above. These regions are shown in **diagram 29**. The vertical column 'A' and 'B' extends for a considerable distance both above and below the set and penetrates floors and ceilings. Anyone sitting, working or sleeping in front, behind, to the left or right of an active cathode ray tube will not be in the strong influence of this vortex field. Anyone directly above or below, however, will be within the core of this field, with the result that the vibrations carried by it will be transferred to their body tissues mainly through the movement of their blood. This is a common situation in offices and blocks of flats.

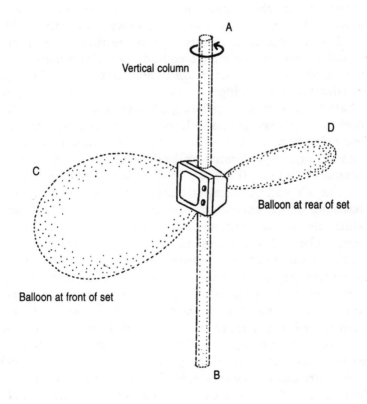

Diagram 29: Zones of disturbance around a television set

The two regions 'C' and 'D' extend for a limited distance in front of and behind the set. Both of these regions have definite boundaries. These are not electromagnetic fields, but regions in which the natural vortices that appear over pathcurve forms are disturbed; this means that water vibrations are disturbed in these zones. The distance these areas extend from the set depends on the design of the cathode ray tube. For a mono-chrome monitor the distance is about three metres, and for a colour tube about eight metres. Since very few people now watch black and white television, and computer operators are always within about two metres, this means that both TV viewers and computer operators are always within this field.

The lap-top, or any other type of computer with a liquid crystal display rather than a cathode ray tube generates only one field from the hard disk, and one from the mains transformer if it is being used from the mains rather than from a battery. The whole operating process from these machines works at a far less aggressive level. The voltages used are only a few volts from a battery or transformer, and there are no cathode rays or vacuums involved. This means about 5 volts instead of up to 20,000 volts needed for a colour monitor.

The TV and the computer are very complex and powerful machines which generate a spectrum of fields and vibrations which are not in harmony with the life forces of the human being. These disturbances all arise as a by-product of the electrical and mechanical design, and are quite arbitrary as far as human physiology and consciousness are concerned. The very long daily exposure times mean that these interferences work on a regular, long-term basis, and as discussed earlier, such chronic exposure to 'noise' can only be harmful to health.

This sort of complex pollution in our environment acts on us in many ways. Some are physiological, such as becoming tired more quickly, or eyestrain. Others are more subtle but no less real, such as addiction to watching the screen. These vibrating fields inhibit the flow of of our life energy. Such interference in the more subtle aspects of our life processes is a consequence of our use of these machines. What, then, can be done about it? The question of protection is of critical importance, and the subject of the last chapter.

---

1 Edwards L., 1993, *The Vortex of Life*, Floris Books, Edinburgh

Chapter 9:
Creating Protective Fields

Since we are surrounded for a large part of our lives by electric and magnetic fields which cannot be eliminated, the question of protection naturally arises. The previous chapters have described situations and processes involved in the relation of water to the new electromagnetic environment. If, as the evidence shows, this environment can cause us problems, then from a practical point of view we need to be able to do something about it. This question has occupied us for several years and the solutions that we have found use new technology which has grown out of a detailed understanding of the vibrational properties of water that have been discussed in the previous chapters. The applications fall into two main areas: one concerns the external environment and the other the interior of buildings.

One of the first indicators of the effect of electricity on plants came to us from the dedicated work of Lawrence Edwards, whom we mentioned earlier. He is an exceptionally accurate observer of the world around him, and has spent half his life-time studying the form of plants and other living organisms.

He is a mathematician and brings all the rigour of a mathematical training to his work on the form of plants. One area of his observation has been the form of leaf- and flower-buds of trees and wild flowers. He has worked on the west coast of Scotland for many years and built up an impressive record of the way in which plant buds change their form. This has given rise to several discoveries.

Earlier we discussed the critical importance of the pathcurve form in nature as a generator of energy vortices over forms. Lawrence Edwards' work has centred on a study of the pathcurve, and has discovered and confirmed the very widespread occurrence of this form in the living world. He has studied many species of tree leaf-buds over the winter months when they appear to be dormant, and made a very significant discovery. The beech tree, for example, has a very slender pointed bud about a centimetre long, which appears to be dormant from October to March, when it swells and sprouts forth the new season's leaves. By photographing one bud every day over the winter, Lawrence has found that the form in fact varies; although it always retains the pathcurve form, the shape of the bud changes. This change goes through a regular fortnightly rhythm right through the winter. The change is small, but quite definite, and has been observed for many winters on trees in a number of different places.

This two weekly variation in the form of the bud appears to synchronise with a particular line-up of the planet Saturn, the moon and the earth. When these three bodies are in line, which occurs every two weeks, then the beech bud changes its shape (**diagram 30**). It is quite a sobering thought to think that all the beech buds on all beech trees perform this change all at the same time through the long cold months of the winter. The same process takes place with other tree species but the planetary alignment is different. The oak, for example, coincides with the alignment of Mars, the birch with Venus, and the cherry with the Sun.

Flower buds, too, follow the same sort of general pattern. The geranium coincides with the lining up of the earth, the moon and Mars, the primrose with the sun and the knapweed with Jupiter. This change in the shape of the plant-buds is a particularly sensitive and accurate indicator of the plant's connection to the planetary rhythms. In 1994 the Schumaker Levi comet was approaching Jupiter on a collision course predicted for mid July. The knapweed is connected to the planet Jupiter, so Lawrence photographed the flower buds of this plant through the flowering season of that summer as he had done for several summers previously. For the whole of the period preceding the date of the impact (which spread out over some time, as the comet disintegrated on its close approach to Jupiter) the knapweed flower buds changed their normal form. They were still pathcurves but different from their normal shape-variations. After the impact, the buds began to return to normal. This is a very remarkable piece of observation: while everyone else's attention was directed upwards to the planet and comet, Lawrence was on his hands and knees watching the direct effect of these events far away in the solar system on a flower-bud's shape.

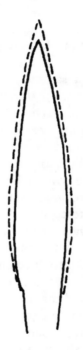

Diagram 30: Fortnightly variation in the shape of a beech tree leaf-bud over the winter months

There appears, though, to be one influence which can change this response of the plant-buds to the planets' rhythms: the presence of electricity. Trees that are close to electric power cables or transformer stations do not follow the planetary rhythms observed elsewhere, and the buds stay more or less the same shape all winter long. The presence of electricity somehow inhibits the change. This is directly connected to the change in the vortex form over the pathcurve described in Chapter 8.

This prompted us to investigate whether there was any way in which trees close to a power line could be protected, which led to some interesting trials. The electromagnetic environment introduces a vibration not naturally present into the water in the tissues of the tree-bud, and this appears to inhibit its form-response. We worked on producing a second set of vibrations that would be strong enough to resist the effect of electro-magnetism. We achieved this by using two elements: vibrations in water, and form.

We imprinted into a sample of water vibrations derived from a number of organic materials such as plant humus. Careful blending of the proportions of these vibrations created a particular pattern of vibrations, or 'piece of music' within the special microstructure of this water. This water was then incorporated into a solid stone pathcurve egg-form, which generates an energy vortex over it. This was done by casting the egg form using the prepared water and ensuring that no unwanted vibrations entered into the process, so that the egg then has the required water throughout its structure, and the vibrations are protected by the calcium carbonate of the solid form. If this egg is placed into the damp soil, then the vibrations from the water spread out for a short distance into the surrounding soil. We found that if a set of three of these eggs is placed in a small triangle in the soil then the effect is very much amplified and the vibrational pattern spreads out for a distance of at least fifty yards (**photograph 2**). In effect a new type of field is generated by the vibrations of the water in the soil, created by the three eggs as a source. We call this a *biodynamic* field, to distinguish it from electric and magnetic fields. This we believe is a new phenomenon, and appears to have considerable potential for counteracting the effects of electromagnetic fields.

These tree eggs have now been in use, in trials on beech trees under power cables, for two years, and the results so far are very encouraging. A set of three eggs has been buried in the soil at the base of a tree that was not responding to the Saturn rhythm due to the presence of electrical vibrations. Over the two years, the presence of the eggs and the field that they generate has rapidly re-established the fortnightly Saturn-responsive rhythm. These tiny egg forms and their biodynamic field appear to affect the form of all the buds on the tree and allow the tree to follow its normal rhythms. This is a remarkable result from something so small, and to a casual eye also very simple. The form, however has to be precise, and the water must carry a complex structure at a molecular level.

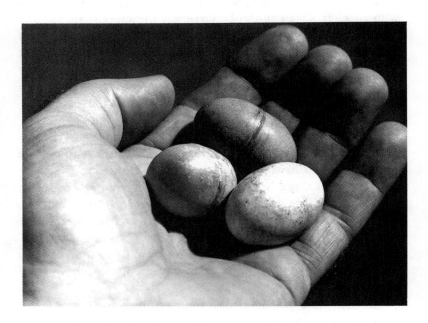

Photograph 2: Set of solid stone egg forms

Vibrating information patterns in water are not very stable. Bright sunlight, freezing, radioactivity and electromagnetic fields all tend to degrade the patterns, and so it becomes necessary to stabilise them if they are to be used effectively and reliably in electromagnetic environments. The way we have done this is to imprint the patterns onto powdered silica. Silica grains are usually covered by a very thin film of water, and a combination of the silica and the water makes a very useful duo on which to store information patterns. If the water on the silica grains is imprinted with vibrating patterns, then they are very stable and withstand strong electromagnetic fields without the pattern becoming degraded.

Silica, therefore, can act as a stable carrying medium for vibrating patterns. It seems at first sight rather unlikely that such a common material should be able to act as a recording medium, when one sample looks and appears to be identical with another. One could, of course, say the same thing about a music tape or a computer disc; they all look identical, and physically they are. At another level they all carry different magnetic patterns which, when activated, transform into music or computer displays of words or pictures. Magnetic patterns are 'read' by machines, patterns on the water of silica are 'read' by living organisms.

It is therefore possible to have a library of information patterns stored on silica in the same way as one might have a library of favourite music on tape. We have three main sources of information patterns: minerals, such as metals and metallic compounds; extracts from living tissues such as plants; and decayed plant material or humus. These three are our basic sources of 'musical elements' for creating new information patterns. From these sources fixed onto silica, biodynamic fields can be created, as we have done with the tree eggs.

In the case of the trees there is only one source of disturbance – the power line and its associated transformers. The process of protection involves strengthening the vibrations in the water of the tree buds and so preventing the vibrations from the electric and magnetic fields having any effect on the water microstructure at a molecular level. This approach is necessary because it is impossible to have any direct access to the electrical system itself. It is important to note that this process of protection does not in any way alter the electric or magnetic fields, but only changes their impact on water.

In the case of a building the situation is somewhat different. The range of electrical equipment is far wider and more complex than the simple power line, but the magnetic machines are not generally as powerful as the distribution transformers. It is also possible to have access to the wiring system itself, which opens up a different approach to the problem of protection. In domestic, office and many industrial situations the main problem is magnetic fields and not electric or electromagnetic fields, because at domestic supply voltage the electric field-strength is usually very low whereas the magnetic field can be quite strong locally. Electromagnetic fields are usually at a very low level unless there is a powerful radio transmitter in the area, or a radio transmitter such as a portable phone is being used.

Magnetic fields can be very intense at the surface of the wire that is causing them, inside an electric motor for example, and also on the wire that feeds the motor. This magnetic field normally sets up a disturbance in any water that it penetrates. We usually think of most things around the house or office as being dry, and in the normal sense of the word this is true. But, as we have seen, virtually everything at room temperature is covered in a very very thin film of water – not in the sense of liquid water that is mobile and free to move, but rather a film stuck firmly to the surface. This is true also for the wiring of the house and the wires inside nearly all electrical apparatus. The water on the wires is exposed to very intense magnetic fields in certain apparatus, and to lower fields in all apparatus and wiring.

All electrical conductors are made of metal and the majority are copper. The metal copper and all other metals are composed of myriads of tiny crystals, and on the outer surface of the crystals of a wire there is a thin film of water. The combination of water and crystals is sufficient for the magnetic field to generate a whole series of column-like vortices along the length of the wire through the vibrations induced in the water. A similar process was described in Chapter 8. This vortex will have an anticlockwise rotation and extend far above and below the wire. In this way the whole wiring system as well as the local coils of wire of electromagnets in particular, generate a complex array of disturbance vertically above and below the system. This disturbance spreads throughout a building having regions of both high and low intensity depending on the distribution of the wiring and apparatus, and when it is on. Fluorescent lights and computers can be on for long periods of time, central heating pumps are usually on intermittently, washing machines are used fairly infrequently. The variation in the use of apparatus and the physical distribution of equipment give rise to a very complex variable pattern of disturbance in any building.

This disturbance is *not* magnetic; it is generated by magnetism, but there is a transfer from the energy of the magnetic field to that of the vortex field, and this spreads far beyond the range of the magnetism. It is because there is water in such close intimate connection with the wiring itself and all the apparatus that this disturbance is generated. In effect the wiring acts as a transmitter of disturbance through the water film upon it. This is of far more concern than the direct effect of magnetic or electric fields on water in tissues, as the strength and extent of a magnetic field in most areas of a building is very low.

In order to provide any protection from this disturbance, it is necessary somehow to have access to the water film on the wires and coils, as this is one of the prime generators of disturbance. Our first attempts to do this followed the same pattern as with the trees, and involved building a biodynamic field using forms and vibrational patterns in water. These met with considerable success but suffered the serious disadvantage of not dealing with all disturbances, particularly those from computers and heavy machines; and also of having a varying effect depending on their position in the building. A much better approach appeared to be to work on the water film directly. In order to do this we had to make a very strong stable vortex with the right vibrational information in it.

As we have seen, water has a microstructure into which vibrational patterns can be imprinted. The microstructures are not all the same and so their properties vary. Certain of these have a property that distinguishes them from all the others when they are imprinted onto silica powder – they can form an energy vortex, even in the absence of a specific pathcurve form. In the case of silica the form is actually in the water microstructure itself. A sufficient quantity of silica made into a compact 'pile' will generate a strong vortex. This vortex can be further amplified by making a triangular arrangement of three such piles as was done with the tree eggs. The result is physically very simple but at a molecular level very complex. This arrangement generates a very strong vortex moving vertically downwards in a clockwise direction. As it passes through the silica it picks up the vibrational information pattern from the water-film on the silica. If a metallic wire is then placed into this vortex, the water on the surface of the wire is set vibrating with the frequencies in the vortex; this can then propagate through the water on the surface of the wire because this water is in intimate contact with the crystal structure of the copper. In this way the vibrations that originate in the water on the silica can be spread down a wire for a distance of at least fifty yards.

The vibration generated in the water-film on the wire in this way is strong enough to prevent any vibration being set up by magnetic fields round the wire. So if the wire is carrying electricity, which means that it is generating magnetism, this magnetism is not able to create the disturbance in the water that it usually makes. *This system completely blocks the anti-clockwise vortex effect of the magnetism.*

If this wire is connected to the wiring system of a house, for example, then the vibrating effect is transmitted to all the wiring and into every piece of electrical apparatus that is connected to it. In this way the negative effect of any magnetic field is prevented at source, i.e. inside the machines and wiring themselves. The magnetic field itself is not affected of course, but the situation is dramatically changed in the water with which this magnetic field comes into contact. In any building there is usually a lot of wire hidden away under floors, in walls and across ceilings so that we live enmeshed in a very complex copper web. If the whole of such a system of wires is set vibrating from a silica source, then the effect spreads out into the space, and any magnetic fields have no effect on any water in this space. In other words, it builds a biodynamic field the size of the building.

Although this is quite a complex process, the end result is very simple. If a **vortex generator is just plugged into the mains wiring, a biodynamic field is set up which blocks the harmful effect that any magnetic field has on water.**

If any piece of apparatus is plugged into an electric socket it would appear to be electrical and therefore be using electrical processes. In the case of the Vortex Unit this is not the case. It makes use of the copper wires of the electrical wiring system, but it does not employ any electrical processes. It uses vibrations in water which are spread by means of the copper wiring, which is quite a different technology and uses principles that are fundamentally different to those of magnetism and electricity.

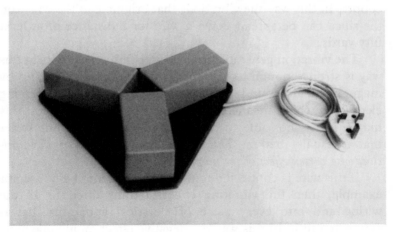

Photograph 3: Vortex unit

This Vortex Unit **(photograph 3)** is now being produced for use in dealing with electromagnetic stress in buildings. One unit builds a field the size of a large house and thus deals with all the apparatus in the building **(diagram 31)**. It was mentioned earlier that disturbances in buildings can come from two distinct sources: those from apparatus and wiring within the building, and those from external sources carried by water in the ground, which appear as a form of geopathic stress generated by heavy magnetic machinery such as transformers. The vortex unit is not only able to deal with disturbances whose source is within the building, but also with disturbances from external sources, which come up from the ground. It seems that this unit is able to generate a biodynamic field strong enough to offer protection from the harmful effects of electromagnetic fields whatever their source.

It is important to realize that creating a protective biodynamic field does not change either the electric or magnetic fields in the area. These are still present and will therefore still register on any appropriate meter. The purpose of the biodynamic field is to change the impact that the electromagnetic fields have on water. One of the commonly reported effects of creating such a field is an improvement in sleep patterns. Disturbed or poor sleep can have a number of causes, which may or may not be linked to electrical or geopathic stress; but removal of these particular stresses can, it seems, help the problem, sometimes considerably.

'Do I have a problem with electromagnetic stress in my house or place of work?'

This is the obvious practical question that people are going to ask themselves. Wherever we use electricity – and there is hardly a building anywhere now that doesn't – we generate some degree of disturbance. So the answer to the question is almost

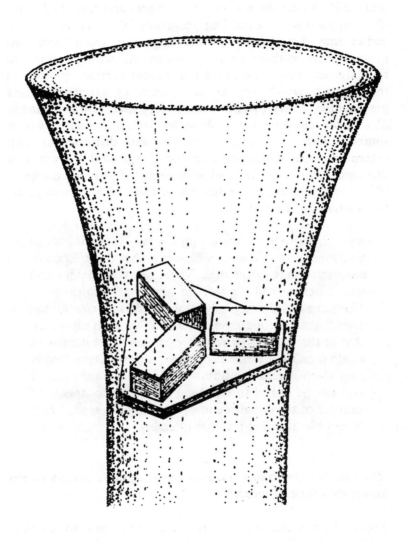

Diagram 31: Energy vortex round a Vortex Unit

certainly yes, to some degree. The level will depend on three main factors;

- the amount of power used
- the type of electrical equipment used
- the presence in the local area of heavy industrial electro-magnetic equipment – particularly transformers

If the level of disturbance is low then we can probably tolerate it just as we can many other environmental imbalances, such as noise or toxins from car exhaust. The point at which we pass from a low level of disturbance that can be tolerated to one that is a potential hazard, cannot be defined exactly for all people since individual tolerance varies for many reasons. Children and infants are much more open and vulnerable than adults, for example, and stress from other factors such as recent illness can lower our tolerance threshold. Most of us would only know when we have reached an unacceptable electromagnetic stress level by the appearance of some form of symptom, although we may not correlate it with this cause. By the time full-blown symptoms appear, it may anyway be rather late in the day to take remedial action.

It is possible to create a protective biodynamic field as we have outlined above. Such a field is a preventative measure rather than a curative one; it prevents the particular stress caused through the effect of electromagnetism on water, and also that generated by geopathic disturbances. Once a stress has begun to have an organic effect in the form of specific symp-toms of illness, removal of the stress factor does not necessarily mean that there will be immediate recovery. The whole concept of protection is to act *before* there is a problem. The generation of biodynamic fields seems to provide a defence against electro-magnetic stress. This work is only in its beginnings, but the results are very encouraging, and it opens up quite a new and different approach to the vexed question of how to live healthily in our very necessary electromagnetic environment, not only within buildings but also in wider external ecosystems.

Appendix 1:
Geopathic Stress

Dowsers and water diviners have long known that underground water has a detectable effect at the surface of the ground. It can only be detected by the human being however – no conventional measuring instruments have been able to register it. Neither, in conventional terms, is there any known way in which water flowing in the ground can create an effect on the surface far above. This lack of explanation and instrumentation has led to the whole subject being largely ignored by scientific researchers in western countries, although the scientific community in Russia has taken it far more seriously: much detailed research has been done there, and some instrumentation has been developed for measuring it. In spite of general theoretical neglect, however, the practical applications of dowsing have been very successfully used by a large number of commercial organisations – a testimony to its reality and to the accuracy and reliability of detection by 'human instruments'.

Earlier this century it was discovered that there are a number of emanations coming from the earth that have quite definite patterns and forms of distribution. Since then, increasing numbers of people have explored this whole area, and a wealth of practical experimental knowledge has been built up. Yet there is a great deal of confusion about the whole complex and rather mysterious subject, compounded by the fact that different people have applied different terminology to the same phenomenon: earth energy lines, black streams, positive and negative lines, polarity, ley lines, water lines, earth energy grids etc.

What is beyond all doubt is that there are widely-distributed patterns and zones of several types of undefined energy at the surface of the earth, of which most people are totally unaware. What is also clear is that these energy patterns are directly connected to substances and processes within the earth, and that they can affect human health.

In the earlier part of this century, Professor Walter, a German doctor, established a connection between the occurrence of certain illnesses and some of these zones of disturbance. He coined the term *Geopathic Stress* for the effects of these zones on his patients. Since then this has been well explored and substantiated by a number of people, some of them from the medical profession. In Germany and Austria in particular, this connection is taken seriously by quite large numbers of people. The fact that most people are either still unaware of the phenomenon or fail to take it seriously does not detract from its reality.

Our researches into the effects of electromagnetism on water, described in Chapter 8, may perhaps be able to throw some light on this subject.

There appear to be five main types of vibrational pattern at the earth's surface which are connected with geopathic stress. Three are natural and two are man-made. These occur in the form of lines of energy varying in width from a few inches up to several yards. Vertically above such lines there is a zone of vibration that affects water. In the case of four of these types, this extends upwards for an indefinite distance, penetrating all materials such as ceilings and floors. The fifth is different in nature, and will be described separately below. In all five cases there are definite frequency spectra within the zones, which can have a direct effect on the water in the human body via the water's microstructure. These frequencies usually act as a disturbing influence – hence the connection with illness.

The first type of natural line is directly connected to flowing water or water surfaces in the ground, which are very common, particularly in certain types of porous ground such as limestone and sandstone. Water surfaces are made in the ground by faults in the rock, which create surfaces into which water can penetrate. The flowing water and the water surfaces form energy vortices above them, not singly but in lines. These are what dowsers and other sensitive people can sense. They have a central core as well as a series of concentric surfaces **(diagram 32)**.

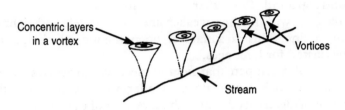

Vortices over an underground stream and the lines that are created by these at the surface. (For clarity, only a few vortices are shown). There exists almost a continuous line of vortices.

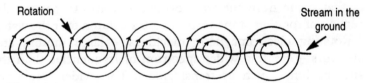

Plan of the above at the earth surface, showing only a few vortices

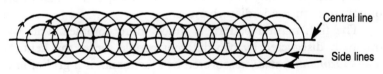

Plan at earth surface showing more vortices and their fusion into lines

Diagram 32: Vortices over an underground stream

These patterns at the earth's surface are formed by all such water situations. Normally these have vortices which are open at the top and rotate clockwise. This direction of rotation and the frequencies carried are not considered injurious to health. They form a network of lines at the earth's surface and constitute many of the earth energy lines. Vertically above such an underground flow there is a line which follows the watercourse, with further, weaker lines to both left and right of the main line. This is a natural phenomenon which has no doubt existed for long ages.

It can also happen that *natural* electrical processes in the earth affect such water flows. Under these conditions the influence of electricity reverses the direction of the vortices, and new, harmful frequencies are added. These are called 'black streams', the second type of energy line **(diagram 33)**.

The third and fourth types of line are very similar to the above, but involve man-made processes. In Chapter 8 we described the effect that a transformer or a power line can have on underground water. The effect of this at the surface is to add strong frequencies that come from the transformer, and also to change the direction of rotation of the vertical vortex column over the water.

Rotating electromagnetic machines – large motors and generators – create a wider spectrum of frequencies than the static machines such as transformers. This wider frequency spectrum is imposed on the water in the ground and propagates as in the third case. This makes a fourth type of disturbance.

The difference between the third and fourth types of disturbance is simply one of the frequency spectrum. Both are of course man-made disturbances.

The fifth natural pattern is much more complex. This was originally discovered by two different people earlier this century. The *Hartmann Lattice*, discovered by Hartmann, is a grid of lines which formed a lattice of squares all over the earth **(diagram 34)**. The size of the squares varied with location, but were approximately 10 square yards. The sides of the squares ran north-south and east-west. This grid has been explored and substantiated by a number of people, and is now a well-established fact.

Appendix 1: Geopathic stress

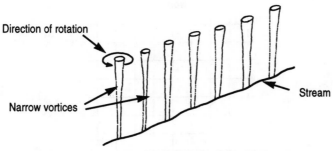

*Vortices and line over an underground stream affected
by natural electricity*

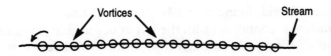

Plan of the above at the earth surface, showing only a few vortices

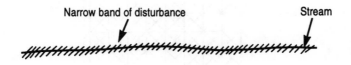

*Plan of stream at ground level showing narrow band of disturbance
caused by many many vortices merging together*

*Diagram 33: Vortices and line over an underground stream affected
by natural electricity*

North

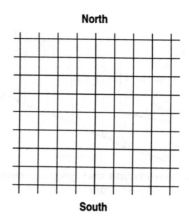

South

Diagram 34: The Hartmann Lattice

A second grid, found by a Mr Curry and known as the *Curry Lattice*, was connected with the layout of the Hartmann Lattice, running diagonally through it in a northeast-southwest and a northwest-southeast direction **(diagram 35)**.

North

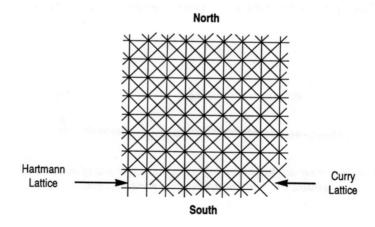

Hartmann Lattice →   ← Curry Lattice

South

Diagram 35: Plan of the Hartmann and Curry Lattices on the ground prior to 1994

These two interrelated lattices formed a complex structure that created narrow lines of disturbance vertically above their location on the ground. As with the other three types of disturbance, these vertical zones penetrated everything, passing through floors and roofs as though they were not there. At the intersection points of these grids were vortices, alternately clockwise and anticlockwise across the grid.

But in 1993/4 this lattice system went through a radical transformation. At Easter 1993, the Curry Lattice disappeared from the surface, leaving only the Hartmann Lattice. The following year, between May and September the Hartmann Lattice broke up and became fragmented, no longer forming a continuous system. Then the Curry Lattice returned in June to rejoin the fragmenting Hartmann Lattice. The result of this transformation is that since September 1994 only the crossing points of the Lattice remain, as a mass of small, quite distinct entities **(diagram 36)**.

These now consist of a series of five, short, narrow planes intersecting each other vertically, which still carry vibrations that can affect water. These forms also all carry an anti-clockwise vortex at their centre. The forms exist at ground level, and at various levels up to about tree-top height. Before the changes occurred, the vibrations from the lattices used to extend vertically above the ground to a great height. This is now no longer the case and they are now only a local phenomenon. To summarise, there are five types of frequency pattern at the surface of the earth:

1. Lines generated by flowing water and water surfaces.
2. Lines generated by flowing water and water surfaces that are affected by natural electricity.
3. Lines generated by water flows and surfaces that are affected by static electromagnetic machinery, such as transformers.
4. Lines generated by flowing water and water surfaces that are affected by rotating electromagnetic machinery, such as motors.
5. Transformed fragments of the Hartmann and Curry Lattices.

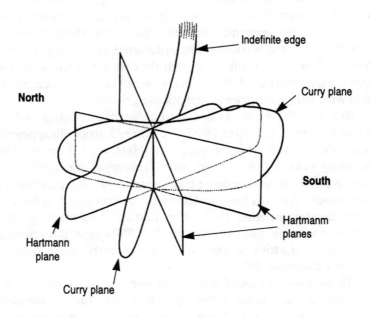

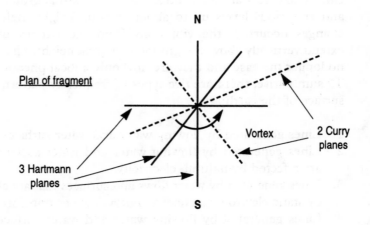

*Diagram 36: Hartmann and Curry Lattice fragment
after September 1994*

All of these are connected with rotating energy vortices, which is how they can be sensed, and each carries a different frequency pattern. Both the vortex and its frequency pattern can affect the water in the human body through the micro-structure of water. Natural, unaffected streams are not harmful to health. In the other four cases, though, the reverse direction of rotation plus the frequencies involved are harmful.

These four sources of disturbance create a very complex pattern of lines and zones over the surface of the earth. We are normally quite unconscious of them, just as we are unaware of the earth's magnetic field. If we spend a fair amount of time in any place that coincides with one of these sources of disturbance, then we are unwittingly exposing ourselves to a health stress, which can have a serious effect over a period of time. Many illnesses, some very serious, have been linked to these disturbance zones. The place where we sleep is one of the most important factors, as we regularly spend about one third of a day there.

The specific correlation of particular illnesses to any one of the above four sources of disturbance has not yet been made, and is a very complicated task to undertake, since there are so many interacting and variable factors.

All such disturbances are often diagnosed in general terms as geopathic stress zones. These are far more wide-spread than is normally recognized, and without doubt constitute a health risk. Surveying and assessing a particular location is best done by calling in someone who knows what they are looking for and how to go about it – not necessarily an easy task. There are various ways in which a disturbed zone can be put right. Some techniques work better than others, and one of the problems is to deal with the wide frequency spectra that these disturbances generate without creating further disturbances.

The remedy that we have explored, of generating a biodynamic field of protection as described in Chapter 9, seems to be a com-prehensive solution to all these different types of disturbance, as well as those created by other forms of electromagnetism, and has grown out of some understanding of how these electromagnetic and geopathic processes work on the microstructure of water.

Appendix 2:
Vortex Structures Over Forms

In Chapter 9 I described the pathcurve form, and the vortex structure over it. In that chapter only one vortex complex was drawn and explained. In fact, the energy vortices over forms can assume far more complicated patterns.

The egg is a conveniently simple form to consider, although what is described below could apply equally to any other pathcurve form.

The set of vortices described in Chapter 8 has a central axis A-B which is vertical, with ten vortice-patterns rising vertically above the egg. This axis also extends below the egg form, with a further set of ten vortices upside down on the same vertical axis. These penetrate the form, meeting and blending with the upper set: the stem of the upside down vortices do not extend above the upper surface of the form.

There are two more axes which carry vortices. These are not in the vertical plane but are inclined at an angle to the vertical as shown in **diagram 37**.

The angles of these two – Y and Z – to the vertical, vary from 0° to 90°, and they are also free to rotate independently, in the horizontal plane around the vertical axis.

On axis C-D there are a further two sets of ten concentric vortices which meet and blend with the upper set on axis A-B. On the third axis E-F there are two more sets of two vortices. The three axes do not quite meet at one point – C-D is always slightly higher than E-F.

The complete picture of the form with its vortices presents a very complex structure, with very subtle and variable dynamics. The axes of C-D and E-F can swing round the

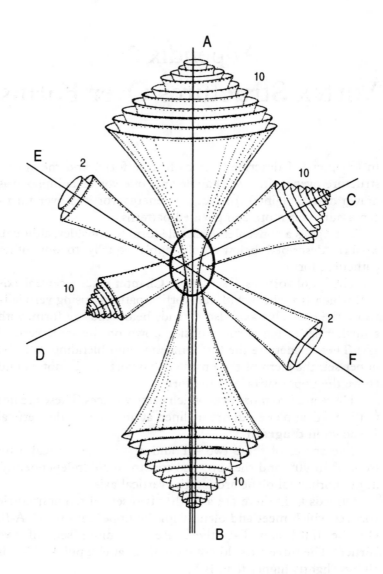

Diagram 37: The vortices around a path curve form

central, vertical axis, in very variable and alive patterns of movement. sometimes swinging several degrees in a minute, and at other times staying relatively static for quite long periods **(diagram 38)**. The movement of these two inclined axes has a dynamic, musical quality, a woven fabric of interpenetrating rhythms. The whole system of vortices and their dynamics goes through patterns of movement that have short, medium and long-term variations. The time of day, month and year, for example, will affect these dynamic movements; they are also related intimately to the movements and relative positions of the planets and stars.

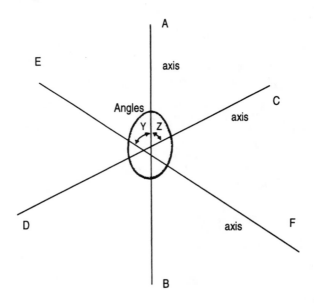

Diagram 38: The three axes of the vortices

These vortices and their dynamics are also intimately related to the water and organic processes taking place inside any living organism. They relate the life forces to the physical substance through the media of form and water.

Glossary

BIOSENSOR
A living organism used as an indicator of change in the environment or in an experiment.

CARCINOGEN
An agent that causes malignancy in living organisms.

CLATHRATE
A cage form of molecules of a substance, which can contain molecules of other substances.

COHERENCE
The existence of definite fixed relationships in time between different waves.

COMMUNICATIONS NETWORKS
Systems of electronic connections over large distances that provide a communication facility.

COUPLING
A connection that exists between two different forms of energy that allows a transfer between them.

ELECTRIC FIELD
A region of space in which electric forces can be detected.

ELECTROMAGNETIC FIELD
A region of space in which there exists a linked combination of electric and magnetic fields (often abbreviated to e/m field).

ELECTROMAGNETIC STRESS
The term used for the harmful effects that electromagnetism has on organisms.

ELECTROSTRESS
The same as electromagnetic stress.

ELECTROSMOG
Colloquial term for the atmosphere of electrical and magnetic radiation harmful to living organisms.

FIELD
A region of space in which a specific energy or force can be found.

FREQUENCY
The rate at which a cyclic process goes through its cycles, usually measured in the number of cycles per second, abbreviated to Hertz or Hz.

GIGAHERTZ
One thousand million cycles per second.

GEOPATHIC
A term used to describe harmful energies emanating from the ground.

HERTZ
The unit used to measure frequency. One Hertz is one cycle per second.

IMMUNE SYSTEM
The automatic response processes of an organism to deal with infection or disease.

INFORMATION PATTERN
A specifically ordered material or energy from which a sequence of data can be extracted to order the sequence of processes.

ISOTOPE
A chemical element having identical chemical properties to another element, but having some different physical properties.

KILOVOLT
One thousand volts. Abbreviated to kV.

LIFE FORCES
Those forces and natural rhythms which orchestrate and regulate biological processes.

MAGNETIC FIELD
A region of space in which magnetic forces can be detected.

MAGNETOPAUSE
The outer boundary of the earth's magnetic field.

MICROSTRUCTURE OF WATER
The very small clathrate forms of which water is composed.

MEGAHERTZ
A frequency of one million cycles per second, abbreviated to MHz.

MODULATION
One frequency superimposed upon another.

MICROTESLA
One millionth of a Tesla, abbreviated to μT

MICROWAVE
Electromagnetic radiation with a frequency in the approximate range 1-300GHz.

MILLITESLA
One thousandth of a Tesla, abbreviated to mT.

MUTAGEN
An agent which causes irreversible cell change in an organism.

PATHCURVE
A line defined in projective geometry, that is invariant in a particular transformation.

PROJECTIVE GEOMETRY
A branch of mathematics taking as its basis the three primary elements of point, line and plane.

RADAR
A radio system using very high frequencies between 1GHz and 30 GHz for detecting metallic objects at a distance.

REGULATION
Control and timing of organic processes.

R.F.
Radio frequency

TESLA
The unit used to measure the strength of magnetic fields.

Bibliography

The following are selected references that are not specifically quoted in the text, but give useful background and detail:

Baris D, Armstrong B G, Deadman J, Theriault G. (1996) 'A case cohort study of suicide in relation to exposure to electric and magnetic fields among electrical utility workers'. Occupational and Environmental Medicine. 53:17-24.

Barnothy M. and Barnothy J. (1960) *Medical Physics 3*. Yearbook Pubs. Chicago.

Bawin S.M. and Ross Adey W. (1976) 'Sensitivity of calcium binding in cerebral tissue to weak environmental electric fields oscillating at low frequency'. Proc. Nat. Acad. Sci. 73 1999-2003. Also Ann. Nat. Acad. Sci. 247:74.

Beale T.L, Pearce N.E. (1995) 'Psychological and physical health correlates of 50Hz magnetic field exposure in humans living near extra-high-voltage transmission lines.' Proceedings of the Bioelectromagnetics Society. 17:87

Beck R. (1978) 'Extremely low frequency magnetic fields and EEG entrainment, a psychotronic warfare possibilty?' Research Associates, LA.

Becker R.O. and Marino A. (1982) *Electromagnetism and Life*. Suny Press, Albany, New York.

Becker R.O. (1990) *Cross Currents*. Jeremy Tarcher, L.A. USA, & Bloomsbury Press, London.

Bennett W. (1994) *Health & Low-Frequency Electromagnetic Fields.* Yale University Press. USA.

Blackman C.F. Benane S.G. et al. (1985) 'Effects of ELF (1-120Hz) and modulated 50Hz fields on the efflux of calcium ions from brain tissues in vitro'. Bioelectromagnetics 6. 1-11.

Blackman C.F. (1988) *Electromagnetic Waves and Neurobehavioural Function.* O'Connor and Lovely, Liss, New York.

Coghill R. (1990) *Electropollution, How to Protect Yourself Against It.* Thorsons Publishing Group, Wellingborough.

Coghill R. (1992) *Electrohealing,* Thorsons.

Coleman M. Bell J. et al. (1983) 'Leukaemia incidence in electric workers'. Lancet 3; 982-983.

Coleman M. and Beral V. 1988. 'A review of epidemiological studies of the health effects of living near or working with electricity generation and transmission equipment.' Intl. Jnl. Epidemiol. 17(1) 1-13.

Coleman M.P, Bell C.M.J, Taylor H.L, Primic-Zakelj M. (1989) 'Leukaemia and residence near electricity transmission equipment: a case control study.' British Journal of Cancer. 60:793-798.

Conti P. Gigante G.E. et al. (1983) 'Reduced mitogenic stimulation of human lymphocytes by extremely low frequency electromagnetic fields.' Diane Publishing Company.

Erren T.C. (1996) 'Association between exposure to pulsed electromagnetic fields and cancer in electric utility workers in Quebec, Canada and France.' American Journal of Epidemiology 143(8) :841

Feychting M, Ahlbom A. (1993) 'Magnetic fields and cancer in children residing near Swedish high voltage power lines.' American Journal of Epidemiology. 138:467-481.

Feychting M, Ahlbom A. (1994) 'Magnetic fields, leukaemia and central nervous system tumors in Swedish adults residing near high voltage power lines.' Epidemiology. 5(5):501-509.

Floderus B. (1993) 'A review of occupational exposure to magnetic fields in relation to leukaemia and braintumors.' COST 244: Biomedical effects of electromagnetic fields. (Xlll/J31/94-FR).

Goffman J. (1981) *Radiation and Human Health.* Sierra Books, US.

Goldhaber M.K, Polen M.R. et al. (1988) 'The risk of miscarriage and birth defects among women who use Visual Display Terminals during pregnancy'. Amer. Jnl. Ind. Med. 13 695-706.

Gordon Press Publishers. 1991. *Electromagnetic Fields: Physiological & Health effects:* A Source Guide.

Grainger P, Preece A.W. (1995) 'Contribution to personal EM exposure from area distribution systems in the UK.' Proceedings of the Bioelectromagnetics Society. 17:123.

Harvey S.M. (1982) 'Characteristics of low frequency electrostatic and electromagnetic fields produced by visual display terminals.' Ontario Hydro Research Divn. Report No. 82-528 IX.

Hatch M. (1992) 'The epidemiology of electric and magnetic field exposure in the power frequency range and reproductive outcomes.' Paediatric & Perinatal Epidemiology. 6:198-214.

Hollows F.C. and Douglas J.C. (1984) 'Microwave cataracts in radiolinemen and controls.' Lancet, 18/8/1984.

Horton W.F. (1995) *Power Frequency Magnetic Fields & Public Health*. Publ. CRC Press Inc.

Huws U. (1988) 'Visual Display Unit Hazards.' London Hazard Centre.

Japanese General Council of Trade Unions (1985) Miscarriages blamed on computer terminals.' New Scientist 23/5/1985.

Justesen D.R. (1980) 'Microwave irradiation and blood barrier Proc.' IEEE vol 68 i: Jan 1980.

Kallen B. and Moritz U. (1982) 'Outcome among physiotherapists in Sweden; is non-ionising radiation a foetal hazard?' Arch. Environ. Health 37 (2); 81-85.

Knickerbocker et al. (1975) 'Study in USSR of effects of electric fields of power systems.' Power Engineers Society, Spec. Pub. 10, IEEE.

Konig H.L. Krueger A.P. et al (1981) 'Biologic effects of environmental electromagnetism.' Springer-Verlag, New York.

Korpinen L, Partanen J. (1994) 'Influence of 50Hz electric and magnetic fields on the pulse rate of the human heart.' Bioelectromagnetics. 15:503-512.

Kung H-te, Seagle C.F. 1992 'Effects of power transmission lines on property values; a case study.' The Appraisal Journal.

Lancranjan I. Maicanescu M. et al. (1975) 'Gonadic function in workmen with long-term exposure to microwaves.' Health Physics, 29; 381-383.

Larkin R.J. and Sutherland P.J. (1987) 'Migrating birds respond to Project Seafarer's electromagnetic fields.' Science 195: 777-778.

Lester J. and Moore D. (1982) 'Cancer incidence and electromagnetic radiation.' J. Bioelect. 1: 59.

Li D-K, Checkoway H, Mueller B.A. (1995) 'Electric blanket use during pregnancy in relation to the risk of congenital urinary tract anomalies among women with a history of subfertility.' Epidemiology 6(5)485-489.

Lyle D.B. and Ayotte R.D. (1988) 'Suppression of T-lymphocyte cytotoxicity following exposure to 60Hz sinusoidal electric fields?. BEMS 9; 303-313.

Maddock B. and Male J. (1987) 'Power-line fields and people'. Phys. Bull. 38: 345-347.

Male J.C. Norris W.T. et al. (1984) 'Exposure of people to power frequency electric and magnetic fields.' Proc. 23rd. Hanford Life Sciences Symp. Oct. 1984.

McDowall M.E. (1986) 'Mortality of persons resident in the vicinity of electricity and transmission lines.' Brit. Jnl. Cancer 53; 271-279.

McDowall M.E. (1983) 'Leukaemia mortality in electrical workers in England and Wales.' Lancet, i 246.

McMahon S, Ericson J, Meyer J. (1994) 'Depressive symptomatology in women and residential proximity to high-voltage transmission lines.' American Journal of Epidemiology. 139:58-63.

Milham S. (1982) 'Mortality from leukaemia in workers exposed to electric and magnetic fields'. New Eng. Jn. Med. 302; 249.

Milham S. (1985) 'Silent keys; leukaemia mortality in amateur radio operators'. Lancet 1; 812.

Miller A.B, To T, Agnew D.A, Wall C, Green L.M. (1996) 'Leukaemia following occupational exposure to 60Hz electric and magnetic fields among Ontario electric utility workers.' American Journal of Epidemiology. 144(2):150-160.

Modan B. (1988) 'Exposure to electromagnetic fields and brain malignancy; a newly discovered menace?' Amer. Jnl. Indl. Med. 13 635-637.

Moore F. (1977) 'Geomagnetic disturbance and the orientation of nocturnally migrating birds'. Science, 196 682-684.

Myers A. Cartwright R.A. et al. (1985) 'Overhead powerlines and cancer'. Conference on electromagnetic fields in medicine and biology. IEEE Conf. Pub. No. 257 126-130.

National Radiation Protection Board (1989) 'Guidance on Standards'. HMSO London.

Nordstrom S. Birke E. et al. (1983) 'Reproductive hazards among workers at high voltage sub-stations', BEMS 4; 91-101.

O'Connor M. and Lovely (1988) 'Electromagnetic fields and neurobehavioural function.' Alan R. Liss New York.

Olsen J.H. et al. (1993) 'Residence near high voltage facilities and risk of cancer in children.' British Medical Journal. 307:891899.

Perry F.S. Reichmanis M. et al. (1981) 'Environmental power frequency magnetic fields and suicide'. Health Physics 41; 267-277.

Perry F.S, Pearl L. (1988) 'Power frequency magnetic fields and illness in multi-storey blocks.' Public Health. 102:11-18.

Perry F.S, Pearl L. et al. (1989) 'Power frequency magnetic fields; depressive illness and myocardial infarction'. Public Health 103; 177- 180.

Phillips R.D. (ed.) (1979) 'Biological Effects of Extremely Low Frequency Electromagnetic Fields.' Proceedings U.S. Department of Energy.

Pinsky M.A. (1995) *The EMF Book: What You Should Know about Electromagnetic Fields, Electromagnetic Radiation & your Health.* Publ. Warner Books Inc. USA.

von Pohl F.G. (1983) *Earth Currents-Causative Factor in Cancer and Other Diseases.* Freich-Verlag, Feucht.

Polk C. (1986) *Handbook of Biological Effects of Electromagnetic Fields.* Publ. CRC Press Inc. USA.

Poole C, Kavet R, Funch D.P, Donelan K, Charry J.M, Dreyer N.A. (1993) 'Depressive symptoms and headaches in relation to proximity of residence to an alternating current transmission line right of way.' American Journal of Epidemiology. 137(3):318-33O.

Prata R. 1993. 'EMF Handbook: Understanding & Controlling Electromagnetic Fields in Your Life.' Publ. Sams.

Preece A.W, Iwi G, Grainger P, Golding J. (1996) 'Pre- and post-natal depression in proximity to high voltage power lines.' Proceedings of the Bioelectromagnetics Society. 18:6.

Preston Martin S, Navidi W, Thomas D, Lee P.J, Bowman J, Pogoda J. (1996) 'Los Angeles study of residential magnetic fields and childhood brain tumors.' American Journal of Epidemiology. 143(2): 105-119.

Meyers A, Cartwright R.A, Bonnell J.A, Male J.C, Cartwright S.C. (1985) 'Overhead power lines and childhood cancer.' In abstracts of the International Conference on Electric and Magnetic Fields in Medicine and Biology.

Reichmanis M, Perry F.S, Marino A.A, Becker R.0. (1979) 'Relation between suicide and electromagnetic field of overhead power lines.' Physiol. Chem. Phys. 11:395-403.

Renova N.V. (1968) 'Influence on the organism of high voltage power frequency EM fields in hygiene, occupation, and biological effects of RF EM fields'. Moscow.

Rivarde C. (1995) 'Electromagnetic field exposure during pregnancy and childhood leukaemia.' The Lancet. 346:21-32.

Robinette C.D. Silverman C. et al. (1980) 'Effects upon health of exposure to microwave radiation'. Amer. Jnl. Epidemiol. 112; 39.

Savitz D. (1988) 'Childhood cancer and electromagnetic field exposure'. Amer. Jnl. Epidemiol. 128; 21-38.

Savitz D. and Calle E.E. (1987) 'Leukaemia and occupational exposure to electromagnetic fields; review of epidemiological surveys.' Jnl. Occup. Med. 29(1) 47-51.

Serduk A.M. and Serduk E.A. (1989) 'Electromagnetic fields; influence on Population Health condition.' BEMS, Ann. Mtg. Tuscon.

Severson R.K. Stevens R.G. et al. (1988) 'Acute nonlymphocytic leukaemia and residential exposure to power frequency fields.' Amer. Jnl. Epidemiol. 126(1); 10-12.

Sharma H. (1984) 'An investigation of a cluster of adverse pregnancy outcomes and other health related problems among employees working with visual display terminals in the accounting offices at Surrey Memorial Hospital'. Vancouver.

Siekierzynski M. Czerski P. et al. (1974) 'Health surveillance of personnel occupationally exposed to microwaves. 2 functional disturbances'. Aerospace Med. 45(10); 1143-1145.

Slesin L. (1987) 'Can cables cause cancer?' Technology Review Oct. 1987.

Stevens R.G. (1988) 'Electric power and breast cancer; a hypothesis.' American Journal of Epidemiology. 125:556-561.

Sugarman E. (1992) *Warning: The Electricity Around You May Be Hazardous to Your Health: How to Protect Yourself from Electromagnetic Fields.* Publ. Simon & Schuster.

Sulman F. G. (1980) *The effect of air ionisation, electric fields, atmospherics, and other electric phenomena on man and animal.* C.C. Thomas, Springfield, Illinois.

Swartwout G. (1991) 'Electromagnetic Pollution Solutions.' Publ. Aerai Publishing.

Swedish Boards, (National Board of Occupational Health; National Board of Housing, Building and Planning; National Electrical Safety Board; National Board for Health and Welfare; Radiation Protection Institute.) (1996) 'Low frequency electrical and magnetic fields: the precautionary principle for national authorities-guidelines for decision makers.'

Tell R.A. and Mantiply E.D. (1980) 'Population exposure to VHF and UHF broadcast radiation in the United States'. Proc. IEEE 68; 215-221.

Tomenius L. (1986) '50Hz electromagnetic environment and the incidence of childhood tumors in Stockholm County.' Bioelectromagnetics. 7:191-207.

Wertheimer E. (1995) 'Childhood cancer in relation to indicators of magnetic fields from ground current sources.' Bioelectromagnetics. 16:86-96.

Wertheimer N, Leeper E. (1979) 'Electrical wiring configurations and childhood cancer.' American Journal of Epidemiology. 109-273-284.

Wertheimer N, Leeper E. (1982) 'Adult cancer related to electrical wires near the home.' International Journal of Epidemiology. 11:345-355.

Wilson B.W. (1988) 'Chronic exposure to ELF fields may induce depression.' Bioelectromagnetics. 9:195-205.

Wilson B.W, Stevens R.G, Anderson L.A. 1989. *Extremely Low Frequency Electromagnetic Fields: The Question of Cancer.* Publ. Batelle Press.

Other books from Hawthorn Press

Enterprise of the Future
Moral Intuition in Leadership and Organisational Development
Friedrich Glasl

Friedrich Glasl describes the future of the modern organisation as a unique challenge for personal development. Every organisation, whether a business, a school, a hospital or a voluntary organisation, will have to develop closer relationships with the key stakeholders in its environment – its suppliers, customers, investors and local communities. Our consciousness as managers needs to expand beyond the boundaries of the organisation to work associatively with the community of enterprises with whom we 'share a destiny'.

216 x 138mm; 160pp; paperback; ISBN 1 869 890 79 5.

Vision in Action
Working with Soul and Spirit in Small Organisations
Christopher Schaefer, Tÿno Voors

This second edition has been thoroughly revised and updated for the 1990's. *Vision in Action* is a workbook for those involved in social creation – in collaborative deeds that can influence the social environment in which we live and where our ideas and actions can matter. This is a user-friendly, hands-on guide for developing healthy small organizations – organizations with soul and spirit.

235 x 152mm; 256pp; paperback; ISBN 1 869 890 88 4.

171

New Eyes for Plants
A Workbook for Observing and Drawing Plants
Margaret Colquhoun and Axel Ewald

A unique approach to the learning and understanding of plant life evolved from the collaboration of Dr Margaret Colquhoun, a leading holistic biologist and Axel Ewald, sculptor, artist and lecturer. Introducing fresh ways of seeing nature, the authors help the reader to embark on a journey of discovery.

A beautifully integrated publication, with inspiring illustrations and authoritative observations, text and image combine to produce a companion guide to plant growth the year round showing how science can be practised as art and how art can help science.

This book invites us to go on a journey, not simply of the imagination, but also of activity and transformation. The invitation is to reconnect with the living forms around us by looking and doing so that our eyes are opened to the nature of plant life.

Dr Brian Goodwin, Dept. of Biology, O.U.

270 x 210mm; 208pp; colour cover; fully illustrated; ISBN 1 869 890 85 X

Workways: Seven Stars to steer by
Biography Workbook for Building a more Enterprising Life
Kees Locher and Jos van der Brug

This biography workbook helps you consider your working life, and make more conscious choices, at a time of great change in our 'workways'. Background readings, thirty seven exercises and creative activities are carefully structured for individuals or self-help groups.

297 x 210mm; 352pp approx; sewn limp binding; ISBN 1 869 890 89 2.

Orders

If you have difficulties ordering from a bookshop, you can order direct from:

Hawthorn Press
1 Lansdown Lane
Stroud
Gloucestershire
GL5 1BJ
United Kingdom

Fax: (01453) 751138   Tel: (01453) 757040

All Hawthorn Press titles are available in North America from:

Anthroposophic Press
3390 Route 9
Hudson
NY 12534

Fax: (518) 851 2047   Tel: (518) 851 2054